S0-CID-989

DISCARD

GETTING REAL STRATEGIES FOR TEENS IN NEED

I HAVE
CANCER...
WHAT'S NEXT?

ELISSA BONGIORNO

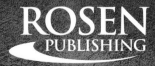

ROSEN
PUBLISHING

NEW YORK

Published in 2022 by The Rosen Publishing Group, Inc.
29 East 21st Street, New York, NY 10010

Copyright © 2022 by The Rosen Publishing Group, Inc.

First Edition

Designer: Rachel Rising
Editor: Greg Roza

Portions of this work were originally authored by Luke Graham and Henrietta
M. Lily and published as *It's Cancer. Now What?* All new material in this edition
authored by Elissa Bongiorno.

Library of Congress Cataloging-in-Publication Data

Names: Bongiorno, Elissa, author.
Title: I have cancer ... what's next? / Elissa Bongiorno.
Description: New York : Rosen Publishing, [2022] | Series: Getting real:
strategies for teens in need | Includes index.
Identifiers: LCCN 2021009418 | ISBN 9781499470666 (library binding) | ISBN
9781499470659 (paperback) | ISBN 9781499470673 (ebook)
Subjects: LCSH: Cancer in adolescence. | Tumors in adolescence.
Classification: LCC RA645.C3 B66 2022 | DDC 616.99/400835--dc23
LC record available at https://lccn.loc.gov/2021009418

Some of the images in this book illustrate individuals who are
models. The depictions do not imply actual situations or events.

Manufactured in the United States of America

CPSIA Compliance Information: Batch #CSRYA22. For further information contact Rosen Publishing, New York, New York at 1-800-237-9932.

Find us on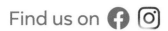

CONTENTS

INTRODUCTION

Being a teen can be a tumultuous experience. Changing bodies and surging hormones can make everything feel seriously out of control. And that's before considering school, friends, and romantic relationship pressure. But sometimes, a much more serious problem can arise. Sometimes, teens can become seriously ill. They can be diagnosed with cancer.

In 2020, about 89,000 young people were diagnosed with cancer, and 9,270 of those patients died, according to the American Cancer Society. Researchers consider "young people" to be ages 15 to 39 years old. Of those young people diagnosed with cancer, 5,800 were teens, ages 15 to 19 years old. In fact, cancer was the leading cause of disease-related deaths for teens ages 15 to 19 with a total of 540.

Statistics like these may be hard to digest. They don't seem real. So, consider the true-life story of Lauren Telesz. When she was 15, Lauren was diagnosed with Hodgkin's lymphoma, a type of cancer that affects the body's lymph nodes. Lymph nodes are glands that help filter out harmful substances. When Lauren was in a children's hospital getting treatment for her disease, there was a playroom for kids younger than her. She didn't feel like she belonged there. A clown visited, but she felt too old for those activities. So she scrolled on her phone and

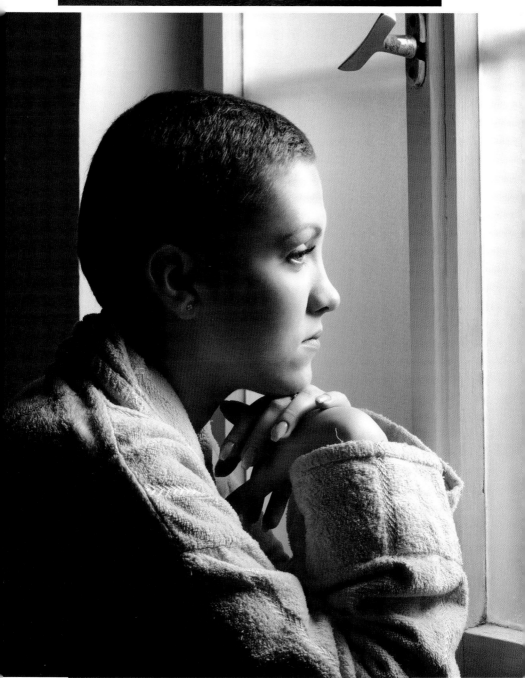

Being sick as a teen can be a lonely experience. While friends are out having fun, you might be stuck inside a hospital trying to get well.

watched her friends getting ready for homecoming on social media. Lauren felt very alone.

But Lauren got better. The five-year survival rate for Hodgkin's lymphoma is very high—97 percent! Once she was healed, Lauren didn't forget that feeling of loneliness. She decided to make a difference. She worked to create a teen center at a hospital in Connecticut for adolescents receiving treatment for

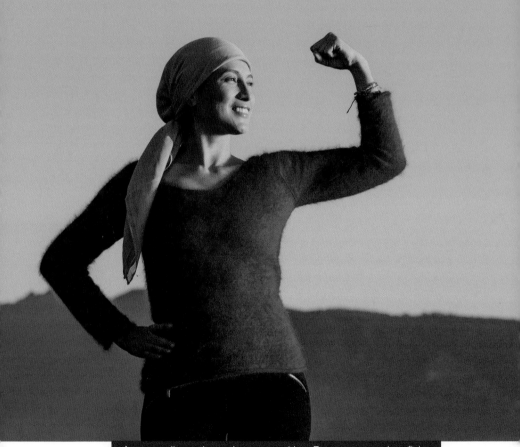

A cancer diagnosis can be a scary thing. But you can work to fight the disease with the help of doctors, family, and friends.

cancer. The center has video games, a virtual reality headset, and other activities for teens.

Lauren's story can provide hope to anyone diagnosed with cancer. She recovered from her illness and was even able to make a difference in other people's lives. It can be very scary to hear that you or someone you love has such a serious disease. However, there are many treatments available for those suffering from cancer. According to the American Cancer Society, five years after being diagnosed, about 83 percent of boys who had cancer and 90 percent of girls are still alive.

A cancer diagnosis can change your life, but it doesn't have to end it. There are many ways to survive and thrive while ill, and after. When facing something scary, it helps to learn more about it. Information is power. This book will help you understand what cancer is, how to prevent it, and what happens after a diagnosis. By learning about cancer, you can be better prepared to help yourself, or anyone else in your life who might become ill.

CHAPTER 1

SO, WHAT IS CANCER, ANYWAY?

There are many different types of cancer. That's what can make cancer so difficult to treat and combat. Some types of cancer can be very deadly. Others have a much higher survival rate. But all types of cancer have some things in common.

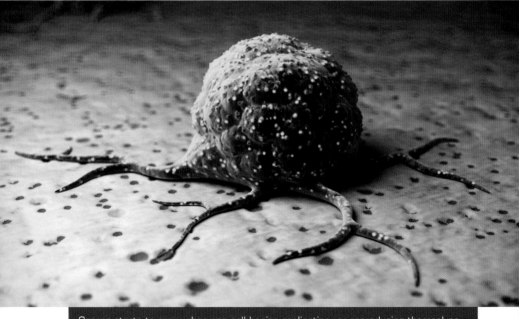

Cancer starts to grow when one cell begins replicating, or reproducing themselves, when not necessary. These abnormal cells grow faster than normal cells.

HOW CANCER WORKS

Cancer begins at the cellular level. That means it starts to develop in the body's cells. Trillions of cells make up the human body. Cells of all different types have different and special jobs to perform.

Every day, the human body experiences wear and tear that damages its cells. New cells are needed to replace old, damaged cells. In order to make new cells, each cell divides in two. Ordinarily, cells divide and produce more cells only when the body needs them. Cells get their directions to divide from genes. Genes control several different functions of the cells. This process of new cell creation and the replacement of old cells is how the human body stays healthy and strong.

Cancer starts when a few cells in the body start dividing out of control. A cancer cell divides even when new cells aren't needed. A cell that goes crazy replicating unnecessarily is called an abnormal cell. Abnormal cells grow more quickly than normal cells. When the abnormal cells keep dividing, a mass of tissue forms. Tissue is a collection of cells that perform a specific function. But the tissue that's formed from abnormal cells doesn't have a function. The tissue made by abnormal, cancerous cells is abnormal too.

The tissue that's formed from abnormal cells is called a tumor. It can grow in any part of the body. Other names for a tumor are growth, lump, or neoplasm. The good news is that not all tumors are cancerous. If you find a lump, talk to a parent and doctor about it, but also know that most lumps aren't cancerous. A noncancerous lump is called benign. So, try not to worry too much and just get it checked out.

IT'S BENIGN!

Benign literally means "to be of a gentle nature," or to be harmless. Benign tumors grow slowly and stay in one place. The cells of this kind of tumor don't invade nearby tissues or organs. They keep dividing and making abnormal tissue, but they don't spread. They keep to themselves. Many of us live with benign tumors or growths without even knowing it. A mole or a wart on your skin is an example of a common benign tumor.

Even though benign tumors aren't cancerous, they can interfere with the normal functioning of the body. Benign tumors may grow large enough to crowd other cells and tissues. If they grow too large, they can be removed, usually via surgery. After removal, benign tumors rarely grow back. Some are completely harmless and thus need no treatment at all. Here are some other types of benign tumors:

• **Abscesses.** These are collections of pus that are usually caused by a bacterial infection. Surface abscesses are called boils. Abscesses frequently occur in moist areas of the body, such as the groin or armpits.

• **Cysts.** These are abnormal swellings or sacs that usually contain fluid. Cysts can occur in almost any body tissue. They are most frequently found in the skin, female breasts, and ovaries.

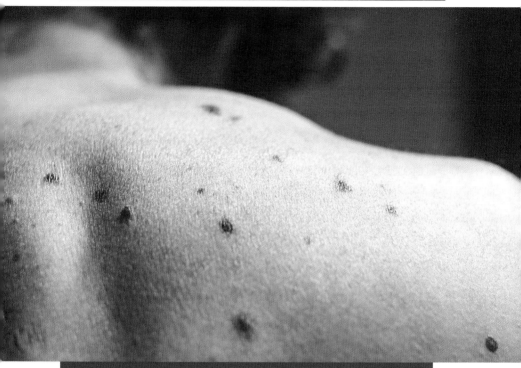

Locating cancerous skin growths early is important because that's when treatment is most likely to be effective. It's a good idea to routinely check your body for new skin growths and changes in existing skin growths.

• **Fibroids.** These are solid growths. They can appear in or around the uterus. Fibroids are made mostly of muscle tissue.

• **Polyps.** These are growths that develop in the lining of certain organs. Polyps may occur anywhere in the body but are most common in the nose, colon, and uterus. They're usually benign, but sometimes a polyp is found to be precancerous, which means that it's in the early stages of becoming cancer.

TO CAUSE HARM

Malignant means "to cause harm." Malignant tumors usually grow rapidly. Malignant cells can invade and destroy nearby tissues and organs. They can also spread to other parts of the body by a process called metastasis. During metastasis, tumor cells break away and form secondary tumors elsewhere in the body. The cells usually travel to other parts of the body by breaking into a blood vessel or a lymphatic vessel. These vessels operate like highways in the body, allowing the tumors to travel and develop elsewhere.

The shape of a malignant tumor often resembles that of a crab, which is how cancer gets its name. The word "cancer" is Latin for "crab." There are more than a hundred types of cancers that can afflict the human body. Most of them belong to one of four major tissue types:

• **Carcinomas**. These develop in the epithelial tissue. Epithelial tissue is the covering of external and internal body parts. Skin is epithelial tissue. So is the tissue that lines or covers internal organs. Carcinomas also develop in the body's glandular cells. Carcinomas are the most common kinds of cancer. They're most often found in the skin, colon, stomach, lungs, and prostate gland.

• **Leukemias**. These are cancers of the blood cells. They are found in the bloodstream and in blood-forming tissues, such as bone marrow and the spleen.

• **Lymphomas**. These are found in the organs of the lymphatic and immune system, such as the lymph nodes, spleen, and thymus. Infection-fighting cells are in almost all tissues of the body, which makes other organs (such as the tonsils or stomach) more vulnerable to lymphomas.

• **Sarcomas**. These develop in the connective or supportive tissues of the body. This tissue includes the cartilage, joints, bones, tendons, muscles, blood vessels, and body fat.

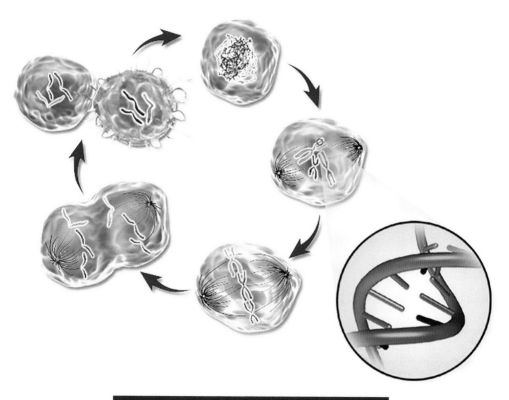

Cancerous cells can replicate quickly. As the cells begin to divide over and over again, a tumor grows.

GENERAL SWELLING

Occasionally, a person may notice one or more swollen lumps along his or her armpits, neck, or groin. These lumps are most likely swollen lymph nodes. Lymph nodes are small, oval structures. They're part of the lymphatic and immune systems. The immune system responds to infections and foreign substances by trapping bacteria and other foreign and invasive disease-causing particles in the

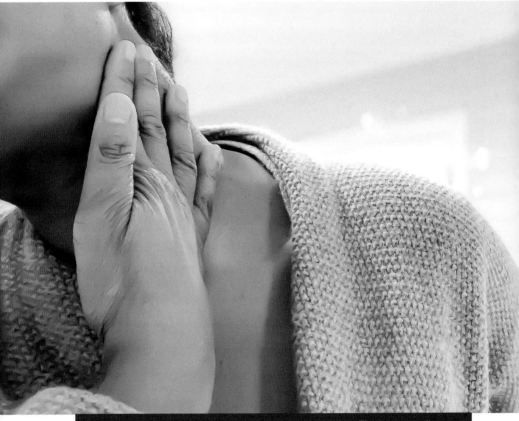

Swollen lymph nodes in the neck can be a sign of infection. They're generally not cause for alarm, unless they remain enlarged for more than two to four weeks.

CANCER 101

It can be scary to think about cancer. But knowing what you're up against will give you the power you need to fight the illness. Be sure to keep these facts in mind when you think about this disease.

• Adolescent and young adults make up about 5 percent of new cancer cases, according to the National Cancer Institute.
• The five-year survival rate for teens and young adult cancer patients is 84.6 percent.
• The most common kinds of cancer in teens and young adults are: thyroid, breast, skin melanoma, and testicular.
• Cancer patients can recover from the disease and live long and happy lives after completing treatment. Many cancer patients can become permanently cured.
• Cancer is not caused by injuries such as bruises or broken bones.
• Cancer is not a punishment or judgment on someone; it's a complex disease. A person doesn't get cancer because of some perceived sin or wrong.
• Pain is not always a symptom of early cancer. This means that feeling pain doesn't necessarily indicate that you have cancer.

lymph nodes. There, they are attacked and destroyed by infection-fighting cells. The lymph nodes swell when they're fighting infection and can feel like lumps just under the skin.

Swollen lymph glands can cause pain and tenderness during colds, flu, ear infections, and sore throats. They can also swell when a person's body is fighting diseases such as mononucleosis ("mono"), some cancers, and HIV infection (HIV is the virus that causes AIDS). To be absolutely safe, any swellings on the body should be shown to a parent, nurse, or doctor.

IMMUNE SYSTEM TO THE RESCUE

The human body works hard every day to combat germs, viruses, bacteria, and parasites. These foreign bodies invade the body because it's a good place for them to grow. But the body has a defense against invaders: the immune system.

Cells of the immune system work to scan the entire body to identify foreign substances. Cells that are natural to the body have molecules the immune system cells recognize. The molecules basically tell the immune system that these substances are part of the body's own cells. The molecules send a "self" signal. An invading infectious substance has foreign molecules the immune system doesn't recognize. These molecules send a "nonself" signal. Immune cells attack anything that sends a nonself signal. The immune system's army of infection-fighting white blood cells moves in to eliminate or kill the intruder.

The immune army is made of lymphocytes and other kinds of white blood cells. These cells are located throughout the body and work together to fight foreign infectious substances. Lymphocytes make substances known as antibodies. Antibodies attack and destroy foreign substances that invade the body.

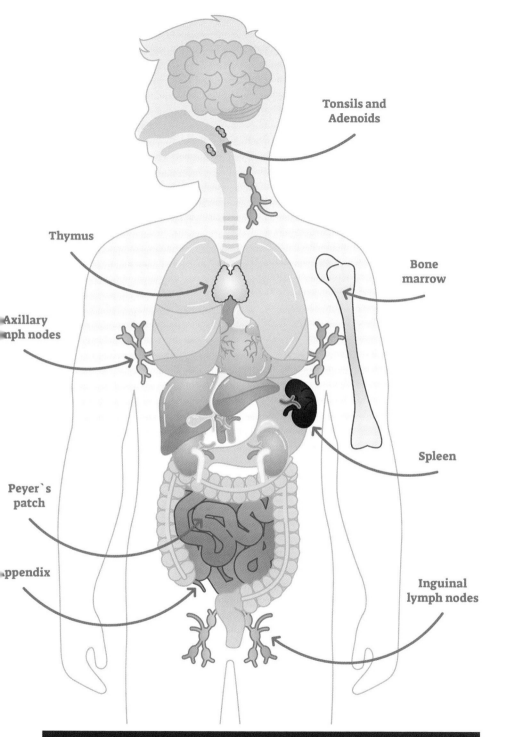

Tonsils and
Adenoids

Thymus

Bone
marrow

Axillary
lymph nodes

Spleen

Peyer`s
patch

Appendix

Inguinal
lymph nodes

This diagram shows the organs and tissues important to the proper functioning of the
immune system, including the thymus, bone marrow, lymph nodes, and spleen. Peyer's
patches are masses of lymphatic tissue found in the small intestine.

ONCOGENES VS. TUMOR SUPPRESSOR GENES

Certain genes are responsible for predisposing an individual to cancer. There are genes called oncogenes, which can help cancer grow. Meanwhile, another group of genes known as tumor suppressor genes can help slow or halt the growth of cancer.

Under typical circumstances, oncogenes play a normal role in cell growth. If the oncogene is altered

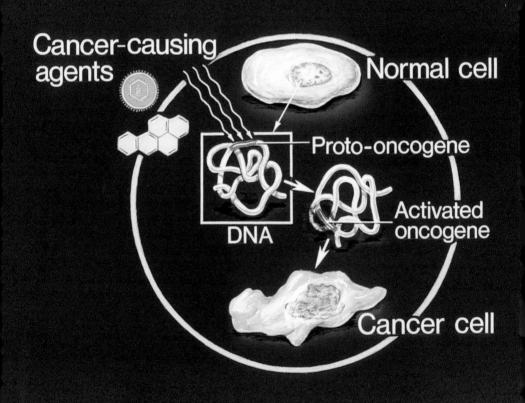

You can see here how a normal cell can turn cancerous when the oncogene is activated. This can be the start of cancerous growths.

in some way, however, or if it appears in high levels, it can aid in the growth of tumors. Indeed, in some cases, oncogenes are normal genes that have been altered by exposure to carcinogens such as radiation and chemicals. In these cases, the oncogene can begin turning normal cells into tumor cells.

Genes instruct the cell in which they reside to maintain the cell's ordinary jobs, such as producing the necessary amounts of proteins or chemicals. If the cell is exposed to radiation or certain carcinogenic chemicals, however, its DNA can be broken or changed. The separated or damaged DNA can then reconnect incorrectly. This forms an altered gene, or oncogene. Once the oncogene has been created and begins sending out its faulty instructions, the cell may produce unusually large amounts of one of its normal proteins or an altered protein. As a result, the cell alters its size, shape, and behavior. It has now become a cancer cell. Cancer cells look very different from normal cells.

When the cancer cell divides, each new cell possesses an identical copy of the problematic oncogene. This means the altered, tumor-promoting gene is already present in the new cells. When these new cells divide, they, too, pass on the same altered, tumor-promoting gene to the next generation of cells. The process goes on and on. As this process of division continues, the rapidly reproducing cancer cells become a tumor. At this point, tumor suppressor genes attempt to do what their name implies: They try to stop cells from growing abnormally. In some

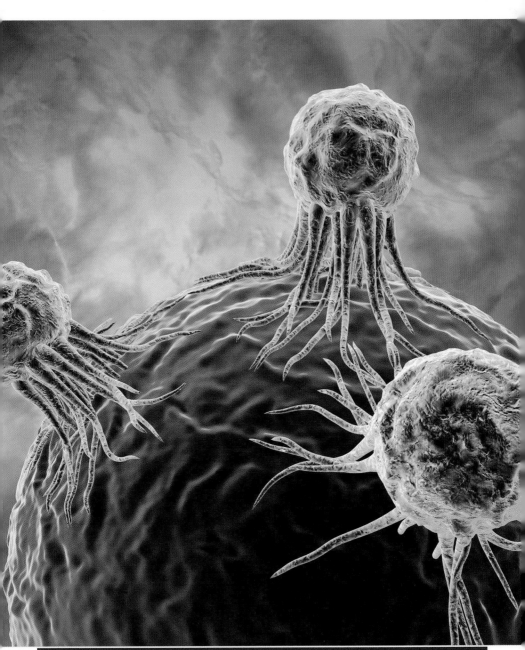

Researchers have found that cancer cells can break away from a tumor and kill specific cells in a vascular wall. They do this to travel to other parts of the body, where they form secondary tumors.

MYTHS AND FACTS

- **MYTH**: If someone in your family is diagnosed with cancer, you'll eventually be diagnosed with it as well.
- **FACT**: Some cancers are passed down through families genetically. But this type of inherited cancer accounts for only 5 to 10 percent of all cancers.

- **MYTH**: Cancer is contagious.
- **FACT**: Generally, you can't catch cancer from someone else. You can still visit and hug someone with cancer. There are viruses, such as human papillomavirus (HPV) and Hepatitis B or C, that can cause cancer. They're transmitted sexually. Hepatitis also can be shared via infected needles.

- **MYTH**: A cancer diagnosis means you're going to die.
- **FACT**: False! The death rate from cancer is declining. Between 1991 and 2017, the cancer death rate decreased by 29 percent. New treatments are being discovered all the time to help cancer patients live long and full lives.

cases, if the tumor suppressor genes are missing or damaged, a cell will continue to grow abnormally and make copies of itself without anything being able to stop it.

CHAPTER 2

WHAT CAUSES CANCER ... AND HOW TO FIGHT IT

Now you know there are different types of cancer that affect different parts of the body. And it all starts with an abnormal cell. Damage or outside influences can cause a healthy cell to turn cancerous. So, what causes that first cell to turn, and how can you prevent it?

CARCINOGENS AND CANCER

A carcinogen is a substance that's known to cause cancer by damaging a cell's DNA. If a person is exposed to a carcinogen over a period of time, they may develop cancer. But this isn't always true. Cancer development depends on a variety of factors, including the health of one's immune system, genetics, and more.

Some carcinogens, such as tobacco and ultraviolet light, can be avoided with a few behavioral choices. People can be exposed to other carcinogens involuntarily through the environment.

Scientists are working to study carcinogens found in the air and water. This can help us to eliminate exposure to dangerous chemicals that could cause cancer, especially in the workplace. As of 2016, the National Toxicology Program (NTP) has a list of 248 known carcinogens. From this list, lawmakers can better understand what substances should be eliminated from use in household products, farming, and manufacturing.

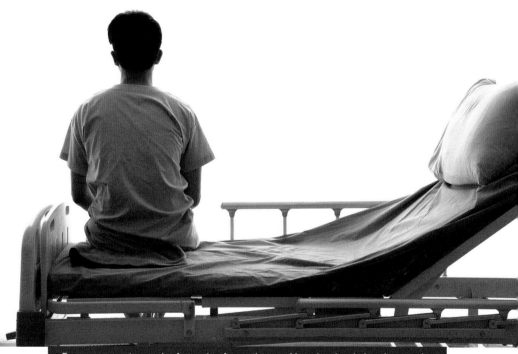

For cancer patients, the future is often unknown. Hope is what helps them endure treatments and personal adversities. Researchers have also given many patients hope as they discover more about cancer—and how to fight it.

TWO PEOPLE: DIFFERENT DIAGNOSES

Certain cancers will begin to grow thanks to a combination of predisposition and exposure to carcinogens. For example, imagine two lifelong smokers. One of the one-pack-a-day smokers developed lung cancer, while the other smoker didn't, even though he smoked the same amount over the same period of time. The smoker who developed lung cancer may have had cells that already had

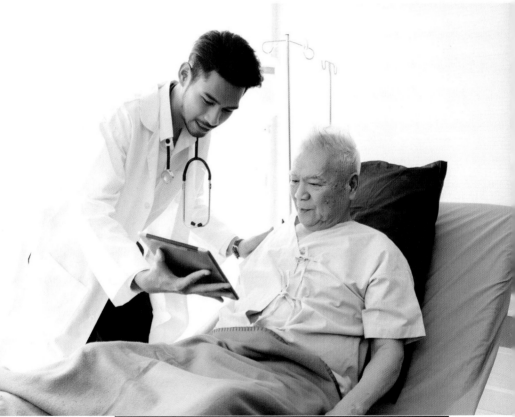

After a cancer diagnosis, it's vitally important for patients to fully understand their prognosis and talk to health professionals openly about the best way to move forward with effective treatments.

a predisposition or tendency to grow abnormally. Under this theory, the carcinogens in tobacco serve as a triggering agent for the cells to become cancerous. This doesn't mean the other smoker was not being exposed to carcinogens. It just means his cells had less of a preexisting tendency to become cancerous.

WHAT CAUSES CANCER?

As researchers study cancer, they know certain conditions and behaviors may lead to cancer.

• **Advanced Age:** Cancer in young people accounts for 5 percent of all cases. The median age for cancer diagnoses is 66, according to the National Cancer Institute. One-fourth of all new cancer cases are found in those ages 65 to 74.

• **Obesity:** Being obese can lead to being diagnosed with cancers such as breast, colorectal, and others. Obesity can also contribute to the severity of illness, including death.

• **Tobacco:** Tobacco, a carcinogen, causes three out of ten cancer deaths in the United States. Nonsmokers exposed to secondhand smoke have a 20 to 30 percent higher chance of developing lung cancer. According to the Centers for Disease Control and Prevention, more than 34 million adults in the United States smoke cigarettes.

• **Alcohol:** Alcohol can increase the risk of cancers of the mouth, esophagus, liver, colon, and breast.

• **Environmental:** About 19 percent of cancer cases come from environmental and chemical causes, according to the National Cancer Institute. Certain jobs are more likely to expose people to these carcinogens, including mining and agricultural industries.

• **Sunlight:** The sun and artificial UV rays, such as those produced by tanning beds, can cause skin cancer.

• **Viruses:** Certain cancers are transmitted via virus, such as the sexually transmitted disease Human papillomavirus.

• **Genetics:** Sometimes the genes passed down from family members can cause cancer.

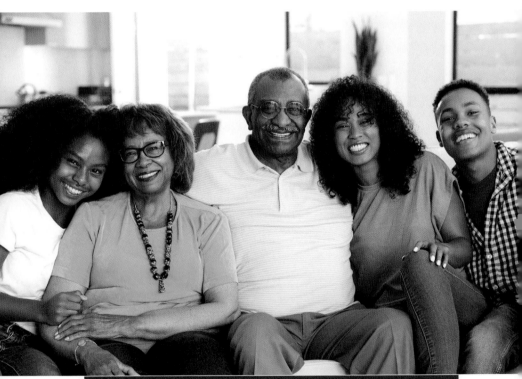

Some types of cancer run in certain families, but most cancers aren't clearly linked to genes people inherit from their parents. Genetic testing may be helpful for those with a type of cancer in their family history, though.

GENETIC COUNSELING AND TESTING

Just because a family member has cancer doesn't mean that anyone related will also get it. Sometimes, family members contract the same type of cancer because they all exhibit the same behavior. They could all work in the same mine and breathe the same carcinogens, for example. Or, they could all smoke cigarettes. But other cancers can be hereditary. In these cases, it can be a good idea for family members to visit a genetic counselor and get genetic testing. Here are some examples of when to see a genetic counselor:

• If a family member had cancer while very young
• If a family member had cancer in multiple organs, such as both kidneys or breasts
• If several close family members (parent, sibling) have the same cancer

A genetic counselor can help families determine if the cancer is known to be hereditary. They will also know if there are genetic tests available to see if the genetic mutation is being passed on. One example of a genetic test is the test for the BRCA gene mutation, which can cause breast cancer. The test for this can let family members know if they are more susceptible to breast cancer.

Remember, just because you have the gene mutation for cancer doesn't mean that cancer will develop. It's important and helpful to know your risk status and to be aware. But many factors contribute to cancer growing, and genes are just one of them.

STAYING HEALTHY

Sometimes people get sick for no reason. However, there are things you can do to reduce the risk of getting cancer. According to the American Cancer Society, about 42 percent of cancer diagnoses and 45 percent of cancer deaths are related to modifiable behavior. That means your actions could save your life. Here are some ways you can make a difference for yourself.

EAT RIGHT FOR LONG LIFE

Eating a healthy diet can help you live a longer and healthier life. It can be helpful to remember to "eat the rainbow" when making healthy food choices. This means eating a range of vegetables that are dark green, red, and orange. It also includes fruits of all colors. Fiber-rich beans, peas, and whole grains are also important. Nutritionists recommend eating five to nine servings of fruits and vegetables each day—in three different colors. By maintaining a nutritious diet, you can stay healthy and prevent diseases.

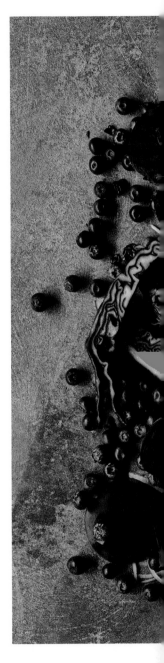

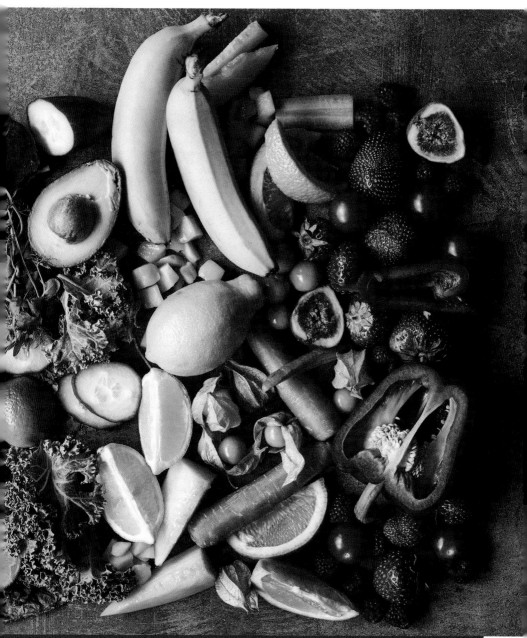

Eating fruits and vegetables in a variety of colors is a great way to get the benefits of many wonderful vitamins. Try some vegetables you've never had before; you might find a new favorite.

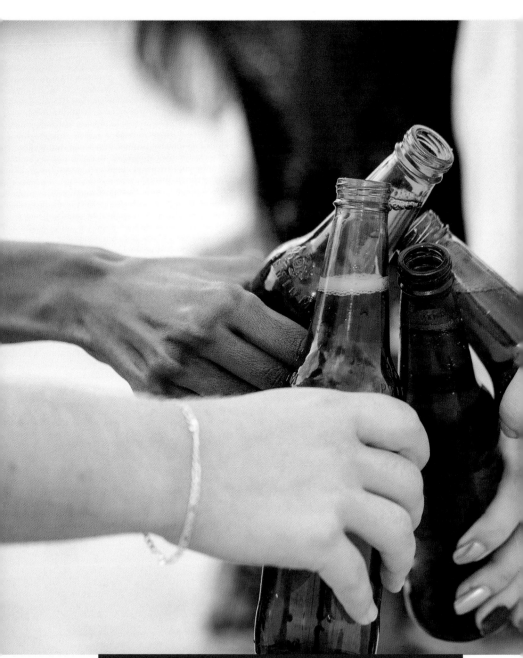

Drinking large amounts of alcohol can cause a variety of health problems, including cancer. Moderation is important when drinking alcohol.

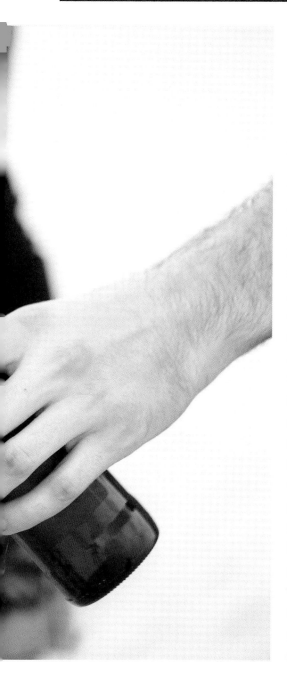

AVOIDING ALCOHOL

Moderate alcohol use is key to the prevention of alcohol-related cancers. Many of the cancers related to alcohol result from heavy consumption. Anyone who develops a dependency on or an addiction to alcohol should avoid it altogether, and anyone who has a family history of alcoholism should consider abstaining. Combining cigarette smoking with alcohol use enhances the cancer-causing effect.

STAY OUT OF THE SUN

Anyone going out in the sun—regardless of whether his or her skin is fair or dark—should use a sunscreen with a high SPF number. "SPF" stands for the "sun protection factor" that blocks both UVA (longwave) and UVB (shortwave) rays. The higher the SPF number, the more protected skin cells are from damage. For a good start toward skin cancer prevention, use a sunscreen with an SPF of at least 15. Some doctors even recommend an SPF of 30 or higher. You can also decrease exposure to sunlight by wearing clothes that cover more skin (including a wide-brimmed hat) and avoiding sunlight from 10 a.m. to 4 p.m.

In addition to seeing a dermatologist for a skin checkup every year, people should perform their own skin checks from time to time. These self-examinations can help you spot any odd changes to the skin, especially in moles or freckles. Get to know how the moles and birthmarks on your body look. As you check your skin from time to time, look for any changes, such as a new mole or skin discoloration, or a sore that doesn't heal. Anytime you see something different, let a parent or doctor know.

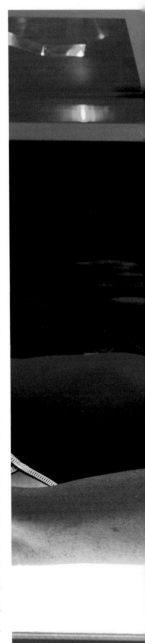

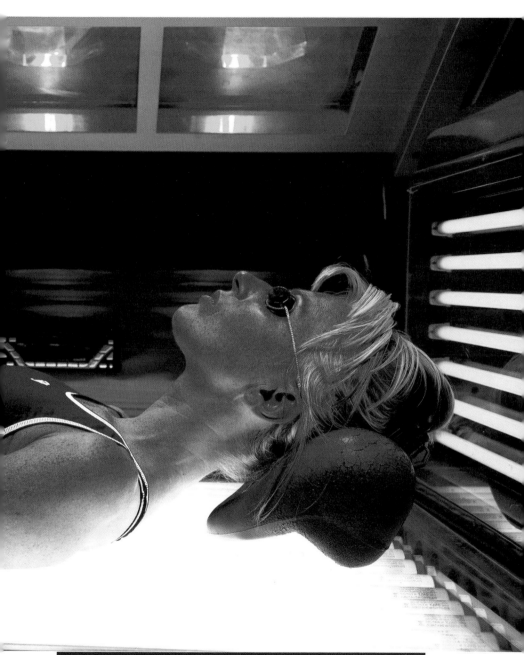

Going out in the sun without sunscreen is dangerous. And tanning beds are an even worse idea. Exposure to harmful UV rays can cause skin cancer.

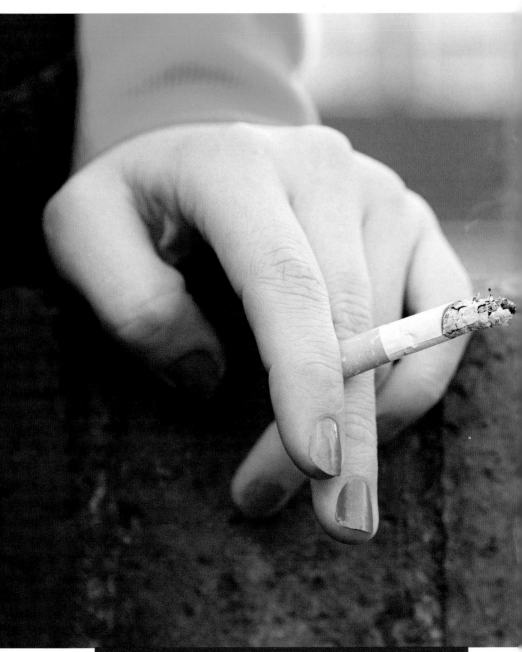

There's no doubt about it, smoking causes cancer. Though hundreds of teens try a cigarette each day, it's a dangerous habit and very hard to break.

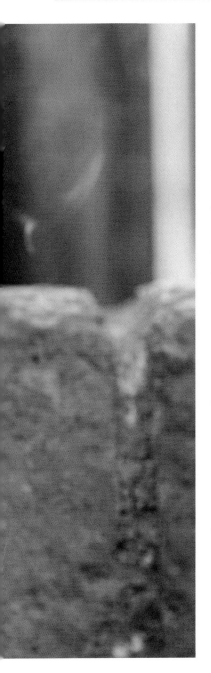

SMOKING KILLS

The effects of smoking are responsible for most cancers of the larynx, oral cavity, and esophagus. In addition, smoking is strongly linked with the development of— and deaths from—bladder, kidney, pancreatic, and cervical cancer. Even though the dangers of smoking are well known, the Centers for Disease Control and Prevention reports that each day, 1,600 teens try smoking for the first time. Smoking is very addictive. You don't want to start; it can be very difficult to quit.

Nicotine patches, gum, prescription drugs, and special counseling programs can help smokers who really wish to quit. There are no good excuses for smoking or for not quitting.

MOVE THAT BODY

Exercise is good for your body for all sorts of reasons. It can help your mental health, and it can help keep certain cancers at bay. The National Cancer Institute suggests a combination of moderate activity, such as a walk, about five hours per week, and more vigorous activity 75 to 100 minutes per week. They also encourage people to include muscle and balance training, too.

It can sometimes feel hard to motivate yourself to exercise, so try inviting a friend along. Check out a new activity, such as Pilates or hiking, and see if you like it. There are also a lot of workout videos online to try. Once you start moving, you may realize you love physical activity.

VACCINES

Imagine being able to defeat cancer with just two shots! The HPV (human papillomavirus) vaccine prevents six kinds of cancer. That's because HPV is a virus that can cause cancer in the vagina, penis, throat, anus, cervix, and vulva. Without the vaccine, 86 percent of people will contract HPV in their lifetime, causing 36,000 cases of cancer each year. But with the two-shot vaccine, given six to 12 months apart, to children starting at age 11, 32,000 cancer cases per year can be prevented.

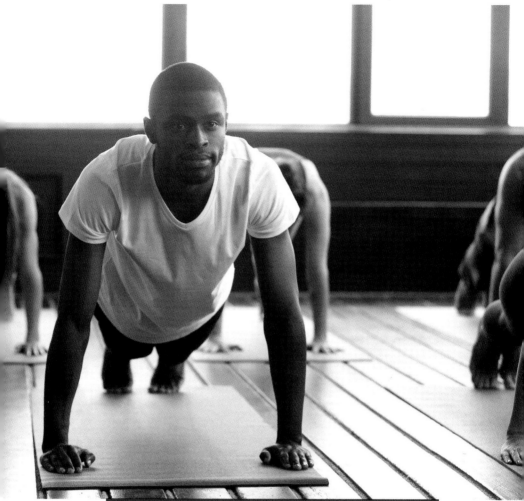

Exercise strengthens the heart and improves circulation. Increased blood flow raises the body's oxygen levels and helps lower the risk of heart disease. Regular exercise can also lower blood pressure.

LEADING A HEALTHY LIFE

There's so much that's known about cancer and its causes. Informing yourself about the causes can help you avoid cancer. By working to prevent cancer you can lead a full and healthy life!

CHAPTER 3

GETTING TESTED

Worrying about one's health can be a nerve-wracking experience. You might feel that something's wrong but you're not sure what. Telling a parent or doctor can be scary, but it's important. It could be that all is well. Or if there's a problem, doctors can help. There are many tests available to discover cancer. And once you know what you're up against, you can fight the disease.

THE ALL-IMPORTANT CHECKUP

It's important to visit the doctor every year. Annual checkups are essential for many reasons, such as an early diagnosis. If a doctor finds any development of cancer early, it can be treated before it spreads to other parts of the body. The earlier cancer is discovered, the better the patient's chances are for recovery and cure. If close relatives have developed cancer, it's important to let your doctor know and then follow his or her advice about cancer prevention and checkups to detect problems early.

For various reasons, the doctor's office is one of the last places many people want to visit. The main reason is that the doctor's office is associated with illness. After all, other than yearly checkups, most people see their doctors only when they're feeling poorly. Getting shots or having surgery at the hospital can be scary too. But the truth is that visiting the doctor, getting shots, or having surgery is a necessary part of maintaining good health.

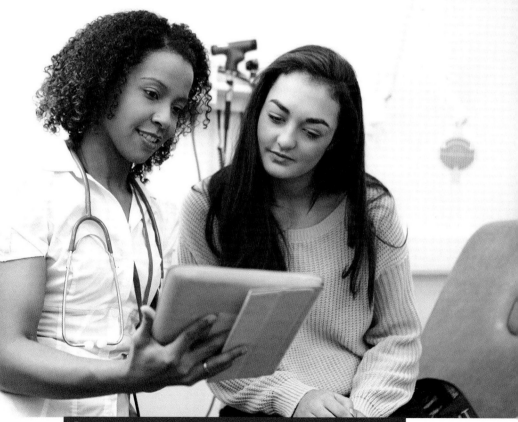

Doctors, nurses, physician assistants, and other health professionals want to help you, so be open and honest about any health concerns you may have and don't be shy about asking questions.

Doctors want us to be healthy. It's their job, their mission, and their passion. Being healthy is a lot more fun and life enriching than feeling sick and tired. And knowing what might keep a person and his or her body healthy is a lot better than not knowing. That's why it's important to think of visiting the doctor as a crucial part of getting better or maintaining good health by preventing illness.

CHECK YOURSELF OUT

You can also keep yourself healthy by giving yourself regular examinations. Checking various parts of the body—such as the skin, lymph nodes, breasts, or testicles—for signs of tumors or other irregularities is an important aspect of health maintenance, cancer prevention, and early diagnosis. This is especially the case for female breast tissue, particularly if a woman has a family history of breast cancer.

Women should check their breasts three days after their period ends (or on the same day every month if they don't menstruate regularly). The self-exam is easiest to perform in the shower. The pads of the fingers should be used to check both breasts for lumps. A woman should start with light pressure and then increase pressure until she gets a good feel for, and sense of, the breast tissue under the skin. The following areas of the breast should be checked:

- Outside: Armpit to collarbone, below the breast, and sides of body
- Middle: The breast itself

• Inside: The nipple area

The breasts should also be examined in a mirror to get a better sense of how they look. This will allow a woman to better notice any sudden changes to them. If a woman notices any liquid coming from the nipples, puckering of the skin, redness, or changes in the size or shape of the breast beyond normal growth during puberty, she should discuss this with a doctor and receive a medical examination. Many lumps and bumps develop in the breast and aren't cancerous. Nevertheless, it's very important to have any lumps and bumps checked by a doctor.

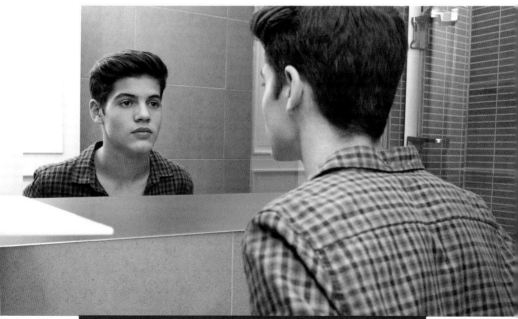

You may wish to ask your physician how to do a regular skin exam, especially if you have worries about skin cancer. If you have a particular area of concern on your body, check it every day for any changes.

WHAT'S UP, DOC?

Aside from your annual checkup, when is it important to go to the doctor? Even if a cancer growth is small, it can cause symptoms. A symptom can tell you something's wrong or different. If you learn to pay attention to how your body feels, you'll know when something has changed or feels off.

Here's a list of symptoms that might be signs of illness. Remember, you shouldn't worry if these symptoms are developing. Just because you experience something on this list, doesn't mean you have cancer. But it's always good to see a doctor just in case. They'll likely reassure you that everything's fine.

- Frequent infections
- A sore that doesn't heal
- Indigestion or difficulty swallowing
- Nagging cough or hoarseness
- Weakness and fatigue
- Loss of appetite and/or weight loss
- Easy bleeding or bruising
- Unusual bleeding or discharge
- Swollen or bleeding gums
- Swollen or tender lymph nodes
- Constant fever or chills
- Changes in bowel or bladder habits
- Obvious change in a wart or mole

TESTING, TESTING

If you go to the doctor and need to have a test for further answers, try not to worry. If you're very nervous, let your parent, nurse, or doctor know.

They can help. There are several types of tests your doctor might administer.

When blood is drawn to test for cancer, a physician or an assistant takes a small sample. The sample is sent to a lab where it can be analyzed. The presence of cancer in the body can cause blood loss, which may present itself as anemia. Anemia means the red blood cell count is low, which the lab analysis will detect. Having anemia doesn't necessarily mean a person has cancer, however.

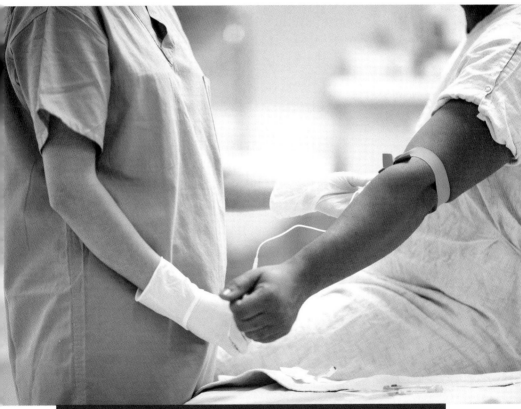

When a doctor is concerned a patient may have cancer, one of the first steps is a blood test. This test can let doctors know what's happening inside your body.

Blood tests can also be used to look for abnormal levels of certain substances. These substances, called markers, can be created by cancer growing in the body. Two kinds of marker tests are CEA and PSA. CEA is the acronym for carcinoembryonic antigen, a substance produced by many types of cancer. PSA stands for prostate-specific antigen, which is produced when the male prostate becomes cancerous.

Urine tests can be used to help determine the presence of cancer in the body. Doctors use a sample of the patient's urine to check for the presence of red blood cells, which can be a sign of illness.

A biopsy is the only sure way to diagnose a cancerous tumor. In a biopsy, the doctor removes a sample of tissue from the tumor or abnormal area. Sometimes, the entire tumor is removed. The tissue sample is looked at under a microscope to see if the cells are normal or cancerous. Biopsies can also show which type of cancer a person has and if the cells are likely to grow slowly or quickly. Biopsies are usually taken while the patient is under a local anesthetic (a numbing painkiller administered to the specific location being worked on). This way the patient doesn't feel any discomfort or pain. A sample of tissue for a biopsy can be removed by surgery or by a needle, depending on the situation.

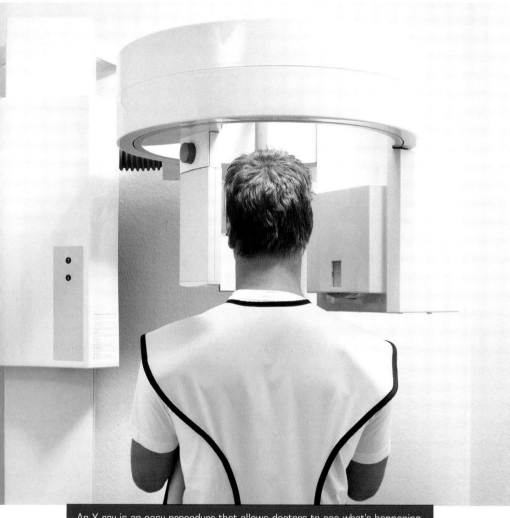

An X-ray is an easy procedure that allows doctors to see what's happening in your body. This is one way to detect if a mass, or tumor, is growing.

IMAGERY

If a doctor would like to see if there are tumors or other growths present, there are many tests they can use. X-rays can provide important clues about the presence or absence of tumors.

If preliminary results suggest the possibility of cancer, the doctor may recommend that the patient undergo a follow-up computed tomography (CT) scan (also referred to as a CAT scan). During a CT scan, the patient lies on a table that slowly slides into a large, tube-like machine. This scan is a type of X-ray that provides very detailed cross-section views of the inside of the body. It can show the exact location and size of tumors. It can also give clues as to the type of tumor and if the cancer is localized or has spread to other parts of the body.

Another type of scan is magnetic resonance imaging (MRI). MRI machines use large magnets and radio frequencies to produce highly intricate views of the inside of the body. The magnet is linked to a computer, which produces extremely detailed images that can be viewed onscreen and printed out.

During a Positron Emission Tomography (PET) scan, a small amount of radioactive tracer is injected into the patient's body. Then the PET scanner can see which diseased cells have absorbed the tracer. This test can see how organs and tissues are working.

An ultrasound diagnostic test uses high-frequency sound waves that can't be heard by humans. These sound waves enter the body and bounce back to a receiver, where they're analyzed. The sound waves' echoes produce an image of the body's interior called a sonogram. The procedure is both painless and harmless. Ultrasounds can distinguish between tumors that are solid (more likely to be cancerous) and tumors that are filled with fluid (more likely to be benign).

An endoscopy is a diagnostic procedure that allows a doctor to look into the body through a thin, lighted, flexible tube called an endoscope. During the exam, the doctor can collect tissue or cells that may look suspicious for closer study. When a specific organ is being examined, the exam is named for the organ. For example, a colonoscopy is an endoscopy performed inside the colon.

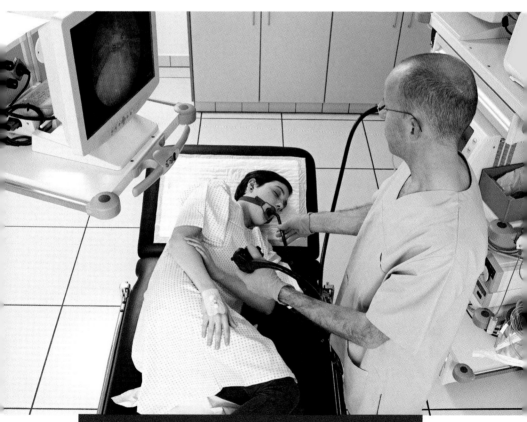

An endoscopy allows doctors a closer look at your organs and tissues. The procedure can also be used to perform minor surgeries, if needed.

A bone marrow sample procedure is performed under a local anesthetic. Bone marrow is the soft, pulpy tissue found within some bones of the body. Tests of the marrow are ordered to determine if a cancer originating elsewhere in the body has spread to the marrow. Samples can also detect cancers of the blood and leukemias. A needle takes a sample of cells or tissue from the bone marrow, usually from the hipbone. The material obtained from the bone is examined under a microscope to determine whether it's cancerous.

A mammogram is a diagnostic test for breast cancer. The breast is placed between two plates that move closer together to compress the breast tissue. Then an X-ray of the breast is taken. Being compressed in this way makes the interior of the breast easier to read on an X-ray. The doctor can see any breast lumps or growths on the resulting image.

A Pap smear test is a diagnostic procedure designed to detect cervical cancer. During a Pap test, samples of tissue are taken from the cervix. The doctor obtains the samples by gently using a small wooden spatula and a cotton swab to collect cells. The cells are analyzed for the presence of cancer.

Bone scans are designed to image only the bones, not the tissues around them. A small injection of a radioactive tracer substance is injected into the patient's arm vein. It travels through the bloodstream and is eventually absorbed by the bones. A special camera takes pictures of the tracer-infused bones. Any dark spots on the bones indicate the lack of absorption of the radioactive tracer and, therefore, a possible lack of blood supply to the bone or a certain type of bone cancer. Especially bright spots indicate areas that have absorbed greater amounts of the tracer, which may indicate the presence of a tumor.

Gallium scans focus on possible cancers of the lymphatic system. A small portion of a metal called gallium is injected into the body. Gallium shows up well on scans. It can give information about the status of any suspicious swollen lymph nodes.

An EEG, or electroencephalogram, is an electrical recording of brain activity. Small recording devices are taped onto the scalp. They record the brain's processes while the patient's eyes are open, closed, and focused upon flashing lights. EEGs are used in diagnosing suspected tumors of the brain.

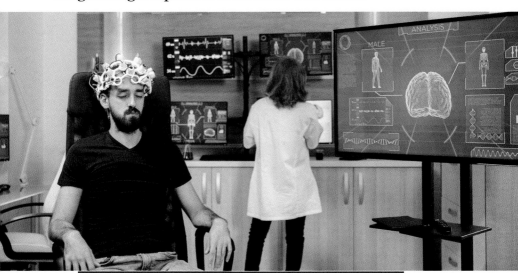

Brain cells communicate with electrical impulses. They are active all the time, even when you're asleep. This activity shows up on EEG recordings as wavy lines. EEGs are safe and painless.

CHAPTER 4

DEALING WITH A DIAGNOSIS

Hearing the words "You have cancer" can be terrifying and overwhelming. Cancer is a very scary disease, and it makes sense that you'd be afraid. But remember, the five-year survival rates for young adults with cancer are over 80 percent. There is hope.

EMOTIONAL OVERLOAD

The emotions experienced by a person newly diagnosed with cancer can be overwhelming. These feelings also can change quickly, often without prompting.

If you've just received a diagnosis of cancer and are feeling out of control, tell someone about it. If it's too difficult to talk to friends or family, you can talk to counselors, nurses, social workers, psychologists, or spiritual leaders. The one emotion that you want to strive for while allowing yourself to feel all the other emotions swirling around you is hope. A diagnosis of cancer is neither a death sentence nor a hopeless situation. Prognosis and survival rates have improved greatly over the years for many types of cancers, and earlier detections have made the fight against cancer far more effective.

For most people, reaching a state of hope is the end result of an emotional process. There are different stages to go through, not necessarily in any order. Sometimes they happen all at once.

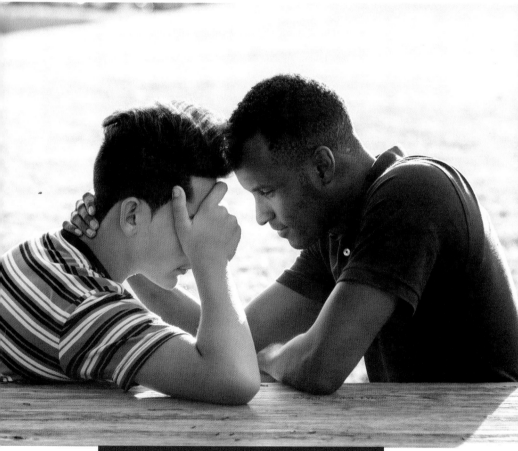

A cancer diagnosis can be a scary situation. Talking with a friend can help you begin to process your emotions.

THIS CAN'T BE TRUE

Denial is a refusal or inability to believe in the reality of a situation. When in denial, you may struggle to make appropriate decisions. Denial is often one of the first responses to cancer. It sounds

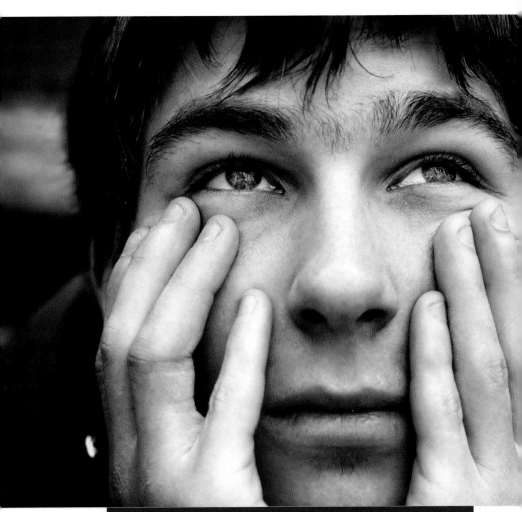

It's very important for someone with a cancer diagnosis to maintain two-way communication with family, doctors, and friends. If you and others express emotions honestly, you can gain strength to deal with the situation.

counterproductive, yet denial serves a valuable protective function. It softens the impact of the diagnosis and allows a patient to adjust at their own pace. It becomes a problem, however, when the patient remains stuck in denial during the time when important and difficult decisions need to be made. While most patients work through their denial, there's counseling available for those who need help doing so.

I'M SO MAD!

Anger is also a very common emotion after a cancer diagnosis. Patients may ask, "Why me?" Remember, cancer isn't personal. It doesn't deliberately and maliciously choose people to victimize. Anyone can get cancer. Good and bad people alike get cancer. People who carefully look after their health and do "all the right things" get cancer, while some lifelong smokers and heavy drinkers may not. Cancer isn't a punishment; it's an illness.

Anger often arises out of feelings that are harder or less "acceptable" to express, such as fear, panic, and helplessness. Being angry can give a person the illusion of being more in control. If you or someone else in your family is experiencing anger, the best thing to do is to try to identify the reason. Try to examine the underlying fear and sadness and make peace with those feelings.

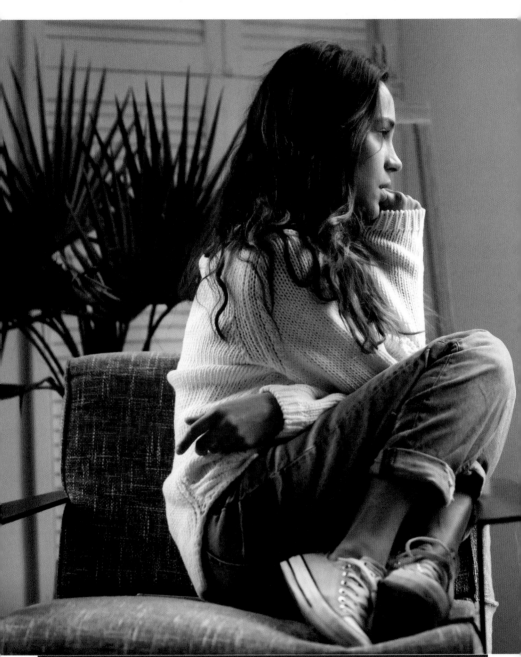

The American Cancer Society's website (cancer.org) has many suggestions and resources about how to deal with a cancer diagnosis. One major piece of advice is to not isolate yourself. It's a difficult time, but you will learn to cope, with the help of others.

I'M SCARED

Fears about cancer often arise because so much is unknown after a diagnosis. You could be scared about pain, side effects of treatment, medical bills and insurance, death, and more. One of the best steps to take toward conquering any fear you may have is learning more about what scares you. Many patients have said that once they learned more about their kind of cancer, they were much less afraid.

STRESS OVERLOAD

The uncertainty following a cancer diagnosis can cause an enormous amount of stress. Stress can reveal itself physically by making the heart beat faster and by causing headaches, a loss of appetite, or dizziness. It also causes sleeplessness and nausea. Stress can weaken the immune system. These are things the body doesn't need, especially while coping with a cancer diagnosis and treatment.

How can you destress? Patients have reduced stress through deep breathing techniques, meditation, exercise, listening to music, reading a book, and talking about it to family members. A quick and easy way to get rid of stress is to take four deep breaths—four counts in, four counts out.

IT'S OKAY TO BE SAD

Some degree of depression is normal when a person is diagnosed with cancer. Patients may experience despair and deep sadness. Depression becomes a problem when it lasts for an extended period or when the patient feels as if there's no longer any point to life. If you've experienced persistent feelings of despair and a lack of interest in your normal activities, and this mood has lasted for at least two weeks without change, tell your doctor. Depression can drain a person's energy, and energy is exactly what's needed most for cancer treatment. Your doctor can give you medication to help you through the depression and can help you get counseling.

IT'S MY FAULT

Cancer patients may feel guilty because they think they've become a burden on their family. They also may feel guilty because they believe their own habits or behaviors contributed to the disease's development. There are support groups that can help everyone in a family deal with the feelings of guilt that arise along with cancer.

FEELING ALONE

No matter how many people a cancer patient has around him or her, being diagnosed with the disease can lead to profound feelings of loneliness. Some friends of the patient won't be able to handle the situation and may distance themselves. Physically, the cancer patient may tire easily and be unable to do all of the things that he or she is used to doing. The person with cancer may feel drained emotionally and not up to socializing. A patient also may have to avoid public places that can be a source of infection.

Treatment is a time to focus on getting better. However, feeling lonely and isolated can weaken the

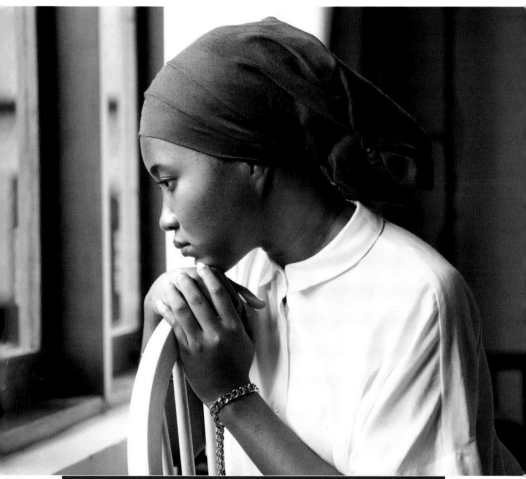

How someone comes to terms with a cancer diagnosis is a personal decision. Choosing whom to tell and whom to ask for support is a part of the process. There's no right or wrong way to do it. Just make sure you reach out.

immune system, which won't be helpful in fighting cancer. In order to fight feelings of loneliness, a patient can talk to other patients in support groups in person or online. It helps to know that others are going through the same things.

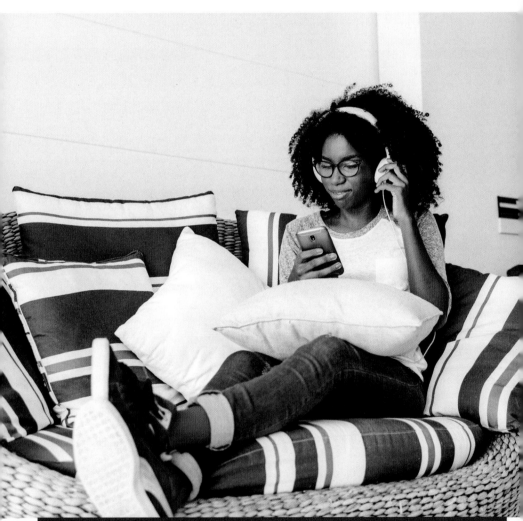

After processing the emotions that come with a cancer diagnosis, it's all right to feel hope. Let yourself believe that you'll be healthy again. The power of positive thinking can make a difference.

THERE'S HOPE!

There are excellent reasons to feel hope, even after a diagnosis of cancer. Modern treatment methods have helped millions of people become cancer survivors. They're now cancer-free. Other cancer patients are living many productive years with their cancer under control in the same way that people with other chronic diseases manage their illnesses. Some doctors believe that if a patient has a strong will to live and a positive attitude, it can make a difference in recovery.

YOU'VE GOT A FRIEND

If you have a friend or family member who's been diagnosed with cancer, it can be a scary time, even terrifying. But you can help. It's okay to be afraid, but remember that you can make a difference in your friend or family member's life. A cancer diagnosis can be a scary thing, but as a friend, you can help lighten the load. Here are some suggestions.

• **BE THERE.** It's natural to be scared of someone's cancer diagnosis, but remember, they're even more terrified. The most important thing to do is to just be there for your friend. Don't avoid them. They're the same person they were before their diagnosis, and you are too.

• **CHECK IN WITH CALLS, TEXTS, EMAILS.** Follow their lead. They may be tired or unable to hang out because of immune issues. If they're not up for a visit, send a card or text a funny meme.

(continued on the next page)

(continued from previous page)

• **LISTEN UP.** After a cancer diagnosis, your friend or family member is working through a lot of emotions. Ask what they need and listen to their answer. If they'd like a visit, you can arrange to stop by. But never visit a cancer patient when you're feeling sick. Their immune system doesn't need to be taxed by a cold or flu. When they talk, don't insist that they'll be all right. Let them have space to discuss their emotions, if they'd like. Or just let them sit in silence. Follow their lead.

• **HELP OUT.** A wonderful thing about friendship is being able to help each other. Ask if you can help with chores, such as laundry or cleaning up around the house. See if they need items from the grocery store, or if they'd like someone to walk their dog. By helping your friend, you're also letting them know you're there for them, which is a powerful offering.

LET'S TALK

One way to deal with a cancer diagnosis is to talk it out. Discussing unpleasant thoughts and emotions can relieve stress and suffering. Getting difficult issues out in the open can be a positive experience because it releases the built-up tension caused by not talking about your concerns. Suppressed anxieties fester and can grow out of proportion to the actual danger of the situation.

There's often a time, in the days after the diagnosis, when cancer patients aren't quite ready to discuss the situation. It's perfectly all right to say, "I don't feel like talking about it yet." But when you're ready, there are options.

WHEN IT'S TIME FOR COUNSELING

Mental health counselors can help you understand, express, and cope with the emotions associated with cancer. The different kinds of community counselors available to you are psychiatrists, psychologists, social workers, and religious representatives. Talking with a mental health professional can be scary at first. But it can be extremely helpful to speak to someone impartial, who doesn't know your parents or your friends. They can see you and any diagnosis from the outside, and therefore offer valuable insight.

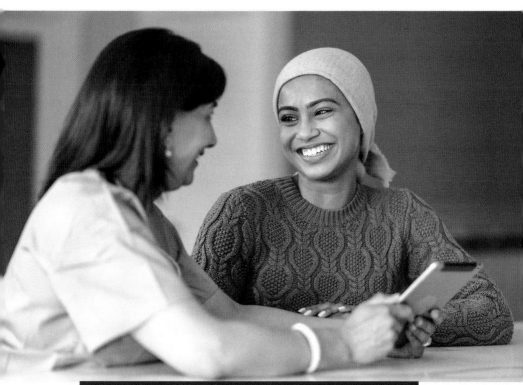

Talking to a mental health professional about a cancer diagnosis can help sort out your emotions. Experts have experience in these matters, and they can help guide you through the scary experience.

If you're having trouble finding a professional to speak with, ask your doctor. They'll have recommendations for you. Let them know how you're feeling emotionally, as this also impacts your physical well-being. Ask a parent to check with your insurance provider to see what mental health services are covered. School counselors also can help find lower cost options if needed. There are resources out there for you; all you need to do is ask.

SUPPORT GROUPS

Sometimes, as a cancer patient, you need to speak to people who truly understand exactly what's happening to you. This is where support groups come in.

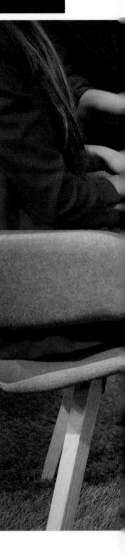

Support groups consist of people going through the same kinds of experiences as you. There are support groups to help cancer patients, some to help families of cancer patients, and others that help both. There's usually a leader of the group who helps guide the meetings. He or she may be a mental health professional (such as a psychiatrist or psychologist) or a cancer survivor. At support group meetings, members can share their experiences, problems, concerns, feelings, hopes, and fears. The other members can offer information on how they dealt, or are dealing, with a similar

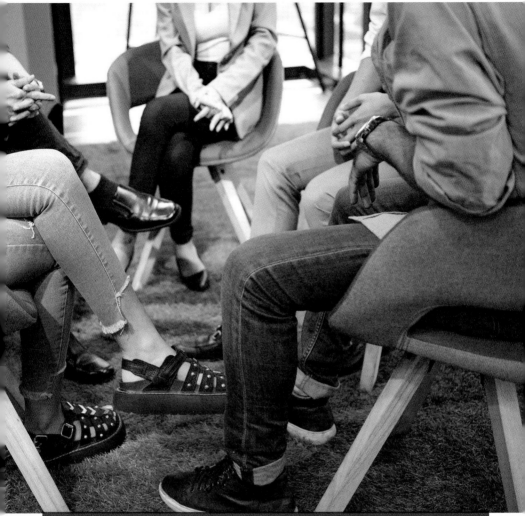

By joining a support group, you can find others experiencing the same problems that you are. They will understand, perhaps better than friends and family, what you're going through.

situation. Members of support groups give each other encouragement, advice, emotional support, and positive energy. Support groups also work to educate patients or family members on advancements in cancer treatment and research.

MOVING FORWARD

As you come to terms with a cancer diagnosis, it's time to start thinking about treatment. Consider composing a list of questions and giving a copy to your doctor. This will allow him or her to answer your questions thoroughly, without getting sidetracked or interrupted. You also can ask permission to tape the discussion so you can listen to it again later at home.

You'll be seeing your doctor often, so there'll be other opportunities to ask for more information. No question is foolish or inappropriate. Also, feel comfortable with asking a question more than once. If an answer to any of your questions is unclear, ask the doctor to explain it in a less complicated way.

Patients can also seek and receive a second opinion from another doctor. This often is advisable because it can reinforce the first diagnosis and treatment plan or offer you alternatives. This is standard practice and doesn't offend your doctor or imply doubt about his or her skills. A satisfactory doctor should be someone who listens to you and takes his or her time with you. You can ask if your doctor is board-certified in a particular specialty. He or she also should know of a good information network for you, which should include access to pamphlets, books, videos, support groups, or counselors. Most important, there should be a positive and creative energy between the two of you, which is an important part of the treatment and healing process.

A cancer diagnosis is a scary thing. But remember to stay hopeful. By talking about your feelings and getting educated, brighter days can be ahead.

QUESTIONS TO ASK A DOCTOR

1. What changes to my body should I be concerned about?

2. What symptoms should I look out for?

3. What type of tests do you suggest?

4. How should I prepare for these tests?

5. When will I know my diagnosis?

6. What treatment options will you suggest?

7. What is my prognosis?

8. What would you do if you were me?

9. What should I do to be healthy and live a long life?

10. What is your best advice for someone to prevent cancer?

CHAPTER 5

WHEN IT'S TIME FOR TREATMENT

After a cancer diagnosis, it's time to work on treatment options. While you deal with emotions, it's also time to get educated. Doctors will help share potential ways to fight the cancer. Then you and your family can decide what course to take.

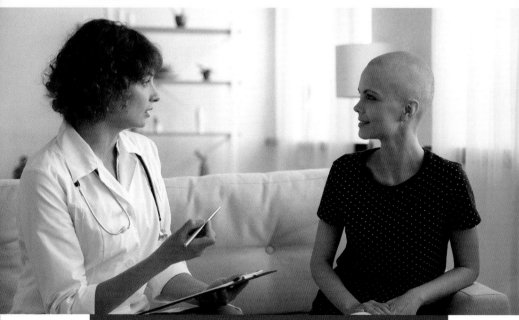

Some people with cancer will have only one treatment to try to rid their body of it. But most people will have a combination of treatments.

STAGES AND MEANING

The stage of cancer describes how extensive the original (primary) tumor is and how far the cancer has spread in the body. If the doctor can't tell immediately, he or she will most likely order tests to determine the stage of the cancer. In some cases, lymph nodes near the tumor can be removed and checked for cancer cells. If cancer cells are found in the lymph nodes, it may indicate the cancer has metastasized, or entered the bloodstream and spread to other parts of the body.

There's no single staging system for all cancers. Some systems cover many types of cancer; others focus only on a particular type. The elements common to most staging systems, however, are:

- The location of the primary tumor
- The tumor size and number of tumors
- The spread of cancer into lymph nodes
- Cell type
- Tumor grade (how closely the cancer cells resemble normal tissue)
- The presence or absence of metastasis

One of the most common cancer grading systems, known as the TNM system, is based on the:

- Extent of the tumor (T)
- The extent of spread to the lymph nodes (N)
- The presence of metastasis (M)

A number is added to each letter (usually I–IV) to indicate the size or extent of the tumor and the extent of spread.

Three common terms that describe how far and to what organs the cancer has spread are "in situ," "invasive," and "metastasized":

- In situ cancer is confined to the place where it started. It hasn't spread.
- Invasive cancer has spread from the tumor to nearby tissues.
- Metastasized cancer has spread to other parts of the body.

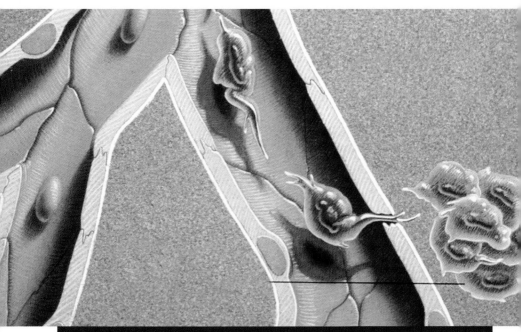

This illustration shows how cancerous cells can spread through the body, or metastasize. The cancerous cells break into the bloodstream with the help of an enzyme.

The grade of a cancer is essentially a prediction regarding whether the cancer cells will grow quickly or slowly. To determine the grade, tumor cells are examined under a microscope in a lab to see how much they resemble normal, healthy cells. A doctor called a pathologist will be able to predict the growth rate of the cancer cells following this close observation.

THE DOCTORS

Patients with cancer often are treated by a team of doctors who are specialists. These are physicians who have highly specific training in a particular area of medicine. Specialists in cancer care include the following:

- **Hematologist:** A doctor who specializes in blood diseases.
- **Oncologist:** A doctor who specializes in treating cancer.
- **Pathologist:** A doctor who specializes in the study of cells and tissues removed from the body (biopsy and surgery).
- **Radiation oncologist:** A doctor who specializes in using radiation to treat cancer.
- **Radiologist:** A doctor who specializes in the making of images of areas inside the body. Radiologists can also explain and interpret the information that comes from the images.

TREATMENT TYPES

There are several different types of cancer treatment aimed at destroying cancer cells. Depending on the type of cancer that is diagnosed, either a single kind of treatment or therapy or a combination of treatments can be used. Treatments can either target the whole body or specific areas.

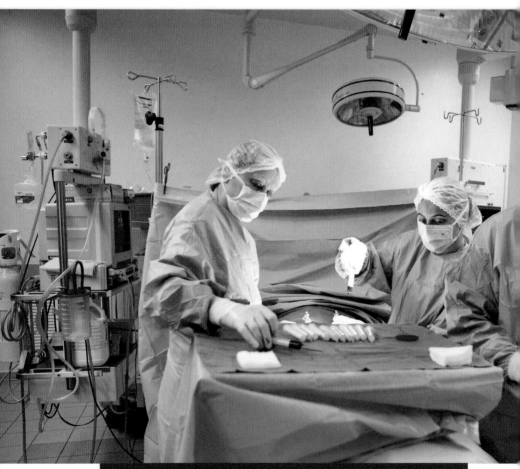

One way to treat cancer is using surgery to remove the tumor. Doctors also may remove tissue around the tumor to try to take out all the cancerous cells.

TUMOR REMOVAL

Surgery is a cancer treatment strategy used to remove a tumor from the body. It's used for cancers that have a low tendency to spread. During surgery, all or part of the cancerous tumor is cut out. Tissues around the tumor and nearby lymph nodes also may be removed. For many solid tumors, surgery is the primary and most effective cancer treatment. A patient may receive radiation before the surgery to make the tumor smaller or make the surgery safer for the patient.

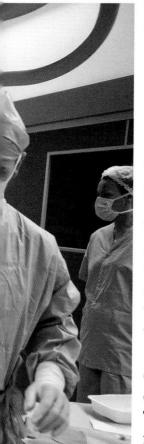

RADIOTHERAPY

Radiation therapy, or radiotherapy for short, uses high-energy rays aimed at cancer cells to kill or damage their DNA to prevent them from continuing to grow and divide out of control. The radiated cancer cells die because they are so damaged they can no longer divide. Normal, healthy cells close to the tumor are also damaged, however, which can make a patient ill.

Radiation therapy is usually given on an outpatient basis in a hospital or clinic five days a week for several weeks. The actual treatments may take only a few minutes each time. The number of high-energy rays used will depend on the individual patient. To make sure

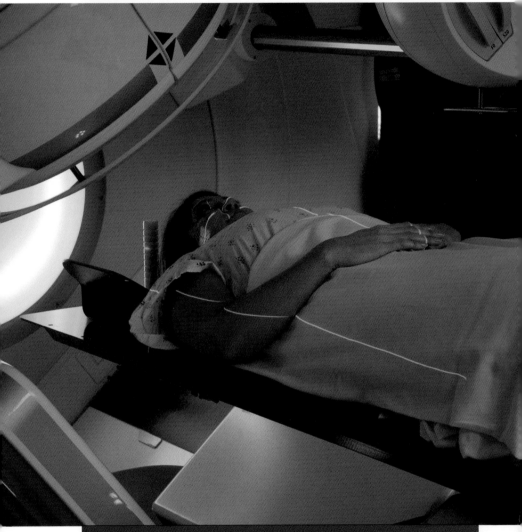

High-energy rays directed at the cancer within the body can work to kill or damage the tumor. The radiated cells will stop dividing, which stops the cancer's spread.

that the rays are aimed correctly and the dosage is appropriate, high-tech scanners are used to create an image of the tumor before each session. This allows doctors to gauge the tumor's current size and location. Then computer programs calculate the required number of beams and angles of the radiation treatment.

The side effects of radiotherapy depend on the part of the body that's treated and the dosage. Some typical side effects are weakness, loss of appetite, and rashes or redness on the skin of the treated areas. Treatment also may cause a decrease in the number of white blood cells, which help protect the body against infection. This means the patient can get sick more easily, so precautions against exposing the patient to germs and viruses must be taken. Although the side effects of radiotherapy can be unpleasant, the doctor can usually treat or control them.

CHEMOTHERAPY

Chemotherapy uses chemicals and drugs to destroy cancer cells. The use of chemotherapy started in the 1940s, when it was discovered that cancer cells became vulnerable when exposed to drug and chemical compounds. Chemotherapy can be used to cure cancer, slow or stop the cancer from spreading, or kill cancer cells that may have spread from the primary tumor to other parts of the body.

Because some drugs work better together than alone, chemotherapy may consist of more than one drug. This is called combination chemotherapy. How often and how long a patient receives chemotherapy depends on the kind of cancer, the goals of the treatment, the drugs used, and the body's response to the treatment. Chemotherapy may be used every day, every week, or every month. It's given in cycles that include rest periods so the body has a chance to regain the strength that's sapped by the treatment and build healthy new cells. Chemotherapy attacks both healthy and cancerous cells, often causing weakness and illness in the patient, so this recovery period is crucial to the treatment's success.

The chemicals or drugs are usually injected into the bloodstream and distributed throughout the body, attacking cancer cells anywhere they're growing. Chemotherapy also can be administered orally (by mouth) in pill or liquid form. It also can be applied topically (onto the skin). When chemotherapy is administered via needle, it can be injected into a muscle, an artery, or a vein (intravenously).

When chemotherapy is given using an intravenous needle (IV), the chemicals drip down from a bag through a tube that connects to the needle. The patient will sit or recline in a comfortable position and remain still while the chemicals are passing from the needle into a vein in the body. When an IV is started, some patients feel coolness or other unusual sensations in the area of the injection. It's important for patients to report any pain, burning, or discomfort that occurs during or after an IV treatment.

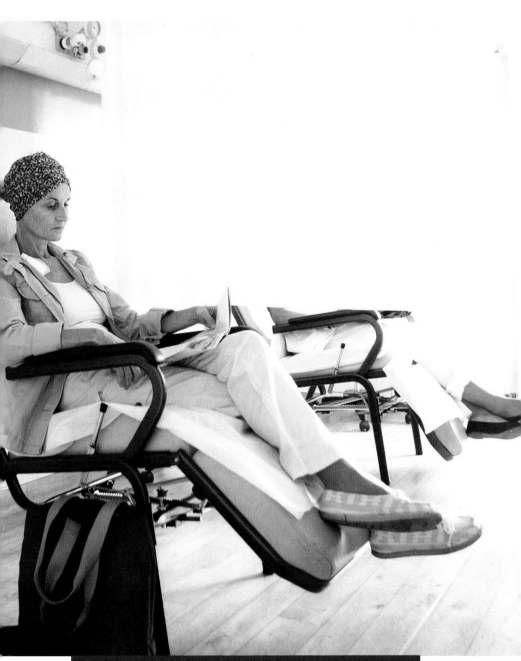

When receiving chemotherapy treatments, some patients read or listen to music or podcasts. Taking your mind off what's happening can allow the appointments to go by more quickly, and with less stress.

Whether or not a patient experiences certain side effects depends on the kind of chemotherapy used and how the body reacts to it. Not every patient experiences the same side effects, and some patients experience few, if any. The side effects of chemotherapy can include nausea, vomiting, hair loss, and fatigue. Other side effects can include an increased chance of bleeding, infection, or anemia. Such side effects occur because, in addition to attacking cancer cells, chemotherapy affects normal, healthy cells. Most normal cells recover quickly when chemotherapy is over, so most side effects gradually go away after treatment is stopped.

One of the largest concerns about side effects is that chemotherapy can make a patient very susceptible to infections. This is because infection-fighting cells (the white blood cells of the immune system) are killed along with cancerous cells during treatment. An infection can begin in almost any part of the body, including the mouth, skin, and lungs.

IMMUNOTHERAPY

Immunotherapy is a treatment that uses the body's own immune system to attack cancer. Biological therapy also can be used to protect the body from some of the side effects experienced as a result of other cancer treatments.

The side effects of biological therapy depend on the type of treatment used and the individual patient. The side effects can include flu-like symptoms such as chills, fever, weakness, loss of appetite, nausea, vomiting, muscle aches, and diarrhea. Other possible side effects are rashes, bleeding, and easy bruising. If the side effects are severe, patients may need to stay in the hospital during treatment.

STEM CELL TRANSPLANT

Stem cell transplantation is the medical procedure that extracts healthy marrow from a donor, harvests stem cells, and injects them into the vein of the patient who has received a dangerously high dose of cancer treatment, such as chemotherapy or radiation. The donor can be a sibling, a parent, children, or even the patient (your own stem cells can be harvested in some cases). A nonrelative who

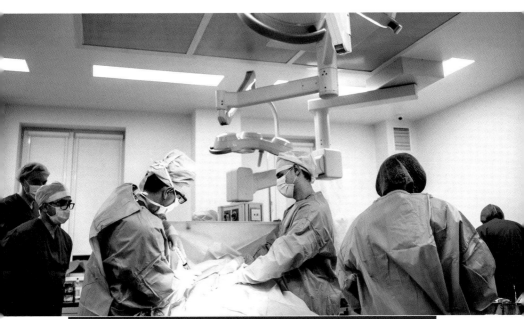

Bone marrow transplants—or stem cell transplants—can benefit people with a variety of cancerous and noncancerous diseases, such as leukemia and anemia. The procedure has some risks as well as benefits.

happens to be a good genetic match also can be a bone marrow donor.

A syringe inserted into the pelvis is used to take stem cells from the donor. The cancer patient is given a dose of radiation and/or chemotherapy and, after some time, is injected with the new stem cells. If the transplant is successful, the patient will be able to receive very high doses of chemotherapy and/or radiation, increasing his or her chances of killing the cancer.

HORMONES AT WORK

Some types of cancer, including most breast and prostate cancers, need certain hormones to grow.

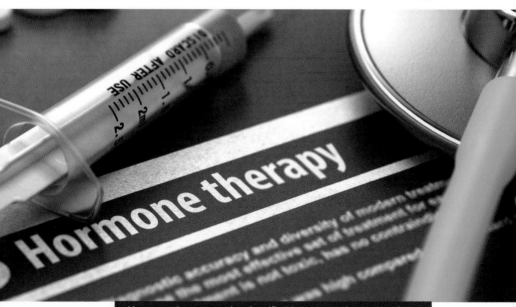

Hormone therapy can be classified into two main groups: those that block the body's ability to produce hormones and those that change how hormones behave in the body.

Hormone therapy keeps these hormones from reaching the cancer, blocking its "food supply." Sometimes, the patient has surgery to remove the organs that make the hormones, such as the ovaries or testicles. Instead of radical surgery, the doctor also can use drugs to stop hormone production or change the way hormones work.

The side effects of hormone therapy can include nausea and vomiting. Hormone therapy also can bring about swelling or weight gain. In females, it may cause hot flashes, interrupted menstrual periods, and loss of fertility. In males, it may result in impotence or loss of fertility. These side effects can be temporary, long lasting, or permanent.

TARGETED THERAPY

Targeted therapy works to control how cancer cells grow and spread via proteins. The treatment plan can use small-molecule drugs that can easily enter cells. Another option is monoclonal antibodies or therapeutic antibodies. These are proteins made in a laboratory. They're designed to attach to cancer cells and mark them so the immune system can attack them. Some proteins make cancer cells stop growing or self-destruct.

There are some side effects from targeted therapy, including diarrhea and liver problems. Doctors have medicine to help.

STAYING HEALTHY

During cancer treatment, your immune system experiences a lot. It's very important to work to keep it strong. When your immune system is strong, the body is better at fighting effectively and efficiently. The immune system is weakened during treatment because infection-fighting white blood cells can be destroyed along with the cancer cells. With fewer white blood cells, the chance of developing infections increases. When the white blood cell count is lower than normal, it's very important to try to prevent infections or lessen their impact. Here are some ways to protect and boost one's immune system:

- Wash your hands often.
- Avoid contact with people who are ill.
- Avoid going to crowded public places unnecessarily.
- Don't take any other medications (including aspirin) or vitamins without first checking with your doctor.
- See your dentist before cancer treatment, rather than during or shortly after.
- Use a soft toothbrush and gentle toothpaste that won't hurt your gums. Brush your teeth and gums after every meal and rinse your toothbrush well after each use.
- Clean any cuts or scrapes immediately with warm water, soap, and an antiseptic (a cleanser that kills germs).
- Use lotion to soften and heal your skin when it's dry and cracked.
- Use protective gloves when doing any yard work or cleaning up after pets.

- Clean your rectal area gently after each bowel movement.
- When blowing your nose, do it very gently into a soft tissue.
- Avoid children who have recently received immunization shots.

By being careful, you can avoid unnecessarily taxing your immune system. This way the immune system can stay strong during treatment.

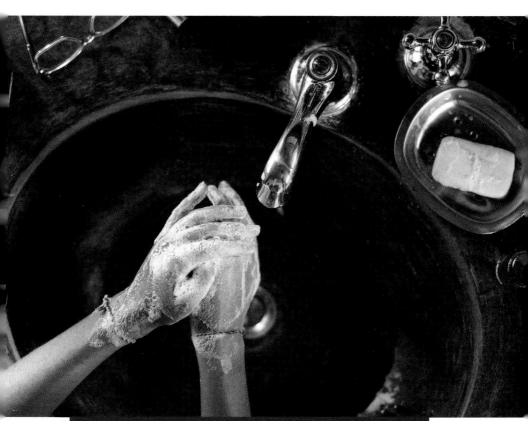

Washing your hands frequently can be an effective way to cut down on spreading germs. You can stay healthy and keep your friends healthy too.

RESEARCH TO THE RESCUE

Clinical trials are responsible for the advancement of cancer knowledge and treatment. They're basically cancer research studies in which promising new treatments are used on humans to make sure the treatments are safe and effective.

In clinical trials, there are strict guidelines for treatment and patient care that must be followed. They require that the doctor make a protocol. The protocol is a plan that explains everything that the study will be doing and why. The plan is then shown to a committee at the hospital or study site. The committee is made up of health professionals, clergy, and consumers. It will reject any protocol that will expose patients to extreme or careless risks.

Once a patient has decided to take part in a clinical trial, he or she must meet certain requirements to qualify. What makes a patient qualified is different for each trial. Some factors that can qualify a person may include age, gender, and cancer type and stage.

The number of patients involved in a clinical trial varies according to what phase it's in. There are three general phases of trials. A Phase I trial is the very first time a new treatment is tested on humans. It usually involves only a small number of patients because the risks of the new treatment in humans are still unknown. Doctors prefer to use patients who can't be helped by other standard treatments. They look for the best way to administer the treatment and watch for any harmful side effects that it produces in humans. Phase II focuses on whether the drug has an

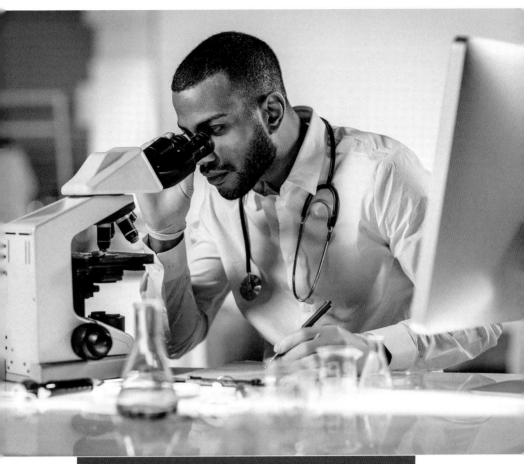

Exciting breakthroughs are happening in cancer research every year. Clinical trials allow scientists and doctors to study potentially life-saving treatments and make sure they're safe and effective.

effect on cancer in humans. Phase III trials include the largest number of patients. Treatments that get to Phase III have shown promise in the other two phases and have caused patients no obvious harm.

There are many treatments to help defeat cancer, and many more are being developed by researchers today. It's important to have hope.

CHAPTER 6

LIFE GOES ON

When you receive a cancer diagnosis, it can feel like time stops. But this is only a temporary feeling. Soon life will be filled with doctor's appointments, treatments, and hopefully, good news.

REMISSION AND TIME

The goal of cancer treatments is to bring you into remission. Remission means that through treatment, the cancer cells and symptoms disappear. When this happens, the cancer is said to be "in remission." Being in remission isn't the same thing as being cured. After remission has been achieved, doctors work on maintaining remission and curing the patient entirely. Remission can last for months or years. If it lasts long enough, the patient is considered cured. The time it takes to be considered cured varies for different cancers. For many types of cancer, a patient is considered cured after being in remission for five years.

IF CANCER COMES BACK

Sometimes, treatments don't work or remission ends, and the cancer begins to grow again. When this happens, it's normal to experience all those emotions again: grief, anger, guilt. When cancer reoccurs, it's not new. It's made of the same type of cells as before. It may be in new areas of the body, but the original diagnosis stands. This means the same treatments may be used again. And the same support system of friends, family, therapy, and more will be needed.

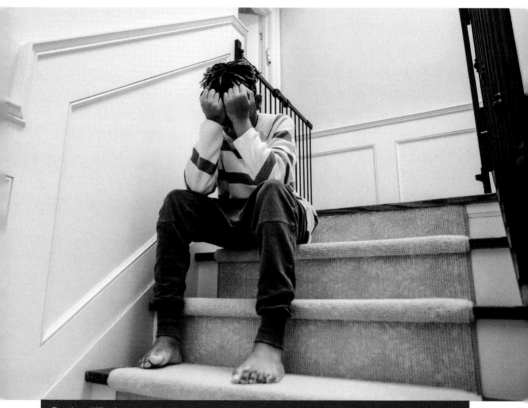

Getting difficult news about cancer returning or being untreatable can be an awful experience. Try talking to a family member, friend, or therapist about what you're feeling.

DIFFICULT DIAGNOSIS

When someone is given a terminal diagnosis, this means the disease can't be controlled, and the patient will die from it. What should be emphasized in cases of terminal cancer is that a prognosis is a prediction. It's an estimate by the doctor on the typical outcome. This prediction is based on the person's age, health, type of cancer, and the stage of cancer and its location. Many people who are given a prognosis of terminal cancer live far longer than expected. Some live to a normal life expectancy, though this isn't typical.

Terminal cancer is commonly referred to as advanced cancer and end-stage disease. People with advanced cancers face many challenges in their daily lives. One recurring challenge is thinking about the future. It can be hard to think of a time when you will no longer be present.

Many patients faced with terminal illnesses come to terms with their emotions by examining their beliefs about life and death. Others, bogged down with anxious thoughts and grief, can lose the will to live. Grief is a normal emotion when dealing with the idea of death, and patients should be encouraged to express their grief any time they experience it. You can try to work through your grief, rather than hang on to it. After grief can come the peace of acceptance or a new understanding of how to live the remaining time in your life.

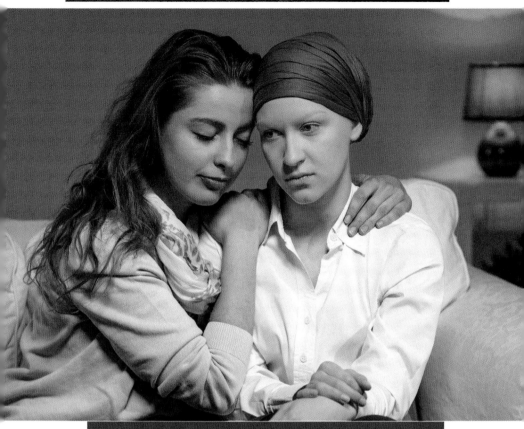

After a terminal cancer diagnosis, a patient will need more support than ever. It will be hard for them to know what to do next, but there are many resources to help them figure out how to proceed with their life.

LIFE AFTER CANCER

When treatment has concluded and a patient is in remission or has been declared cured, some may find they have a new understanding about themselves and life. To have faced such a serious diagnosis and survived, they have a perspective others don't. Many patients have a new zest for life and take more chances than they did before developing cancer. Others try to enjoy and make the most of every moment, such as stopping to take in simple moments, sitting in the backyard and listening to birds sing, or watching dogs play.

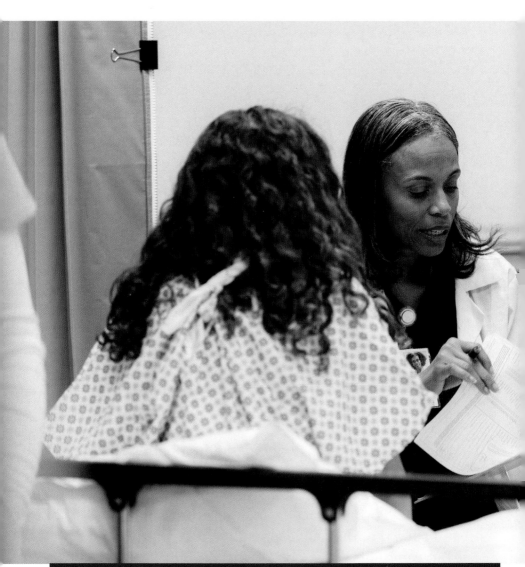

Going to checkups with your doctor after you're in remission can be stressful. Old memories may surface. But remember, staying healthy should be one of your top priorities.

Going through cancer treatment can [...] a person how to take excellent care of his [...] health. Once treatment has brought about re[...]

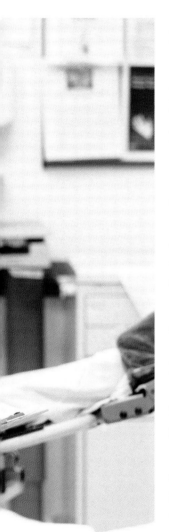

sion, it's important that the pati[...] keep working on maintaining good health. The health needs of a patient in remission differ from person to person. Your doctor will give you an idea of your health needs and what you need to do in order to ensure good health in both the short-term and long-term. These guidelines should be followed closely to ensure that you make the most of your return to health and help prevent a cancer recurrence or development of other diseases or illnesses.

Once you're deemed a cancer survivor, it's cause for celebration! But you must remember that keeping regular checkups, watching for warning signs, and maintaining good health habits are very important. After the conclusion of cancer treatments, patients should see their doctors about every three months. As time passes and the recovery progresses without any recurrences or other health problems, time between appointments may become longer.

WHAT TO LOOK OUT FOR:
STAYING HEALTHY & AWARE

Once you've recovered from cancer, it's still important to pay attention to your body. If one of the following symptoms occurs before, during, or after cancer treatments, be sure to contact a doctor right away.

- A new lump or growth where your cancer first started
- Unexplained weight loss
- Easy bleeding
- Unexplained bruising
- Fever (when the temperature is above 100°F [37.7°C])
- Sweating
- Chills
- Severe coughing or sore throat
- Diarrhea
- Burning sensation when you urinate
- Unusual vaginal discharge or itching
- Redness or tenderness, especially around any wounds, sores, or pimples

If you experience any other side effect or feel out of sorts in any way during or after treatment, let an adult and your doctor know. You can ask for a list of expected side effects, but you know your body better than anyone else. Tune in and speak up.

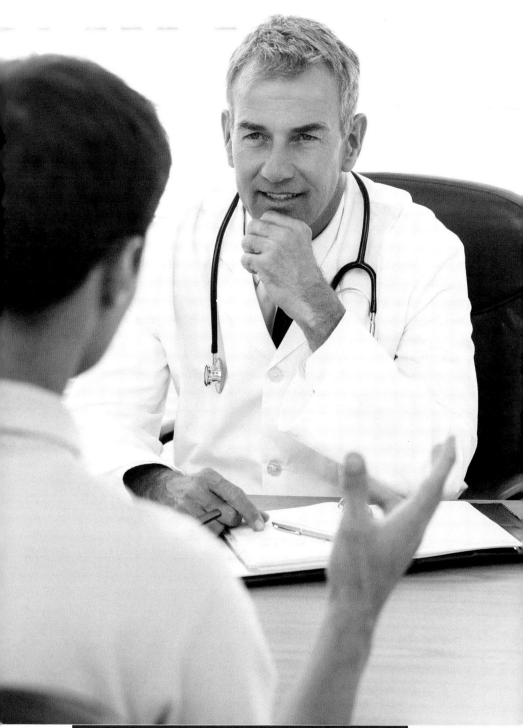

A recurrence of cancer isn't always detected through visits to the doctor. It's often the patient who recognizes something is wrong and who brings the problem to the attention of the doctor.

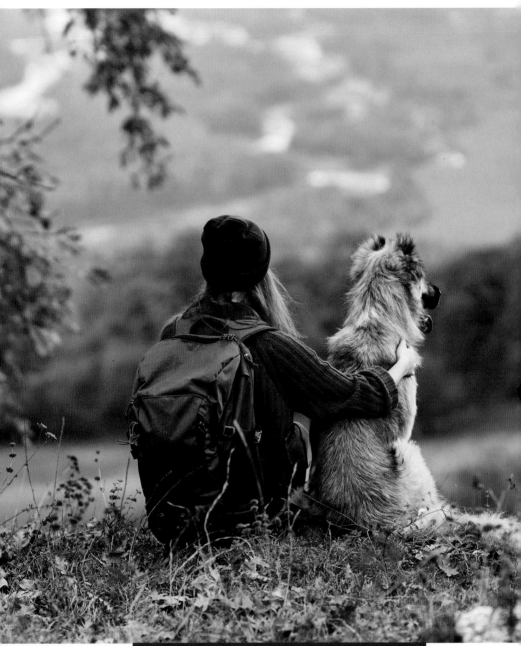

Facing cancer and coming out healthy can be a life-affirming experience. Get out there and enjoy life!

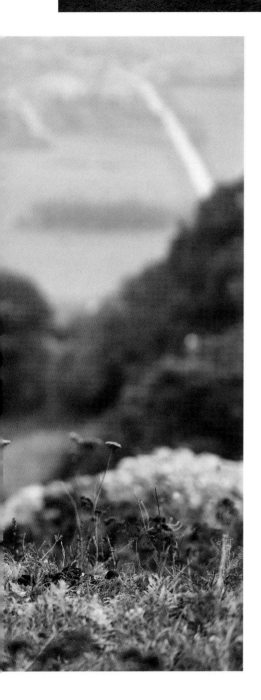

It's completely normal for a cancer survivor to have a lot of anxiety around cancer and illness. Being worried about the cancer returning is an absolutely understandable way to feel. Especially around the time of regular checkups, anxiety could spike. Try using the same tools deployed before and during treatment. Talk with a friend. Take deep breaths. Check in with your therapist. Attend a group meeting and share how you're feeling with other survivors. They can best relate to what you're going through. When you realize you're not alone, your worries might subside.

Surviving cancer is a gift—a gift of perspective, an appreciation for life. While there are worries, there also should be celebration and appreciation, appreciation of yourself and your body. With this newfound perceptive, cancer survivors can choose healthier lifestyles and be thankful for all they have. Life is good!

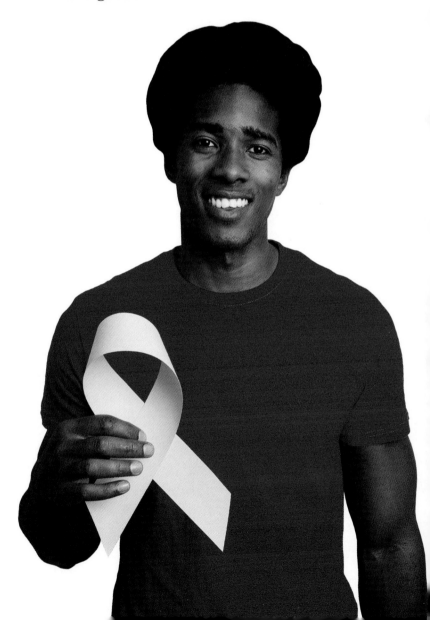

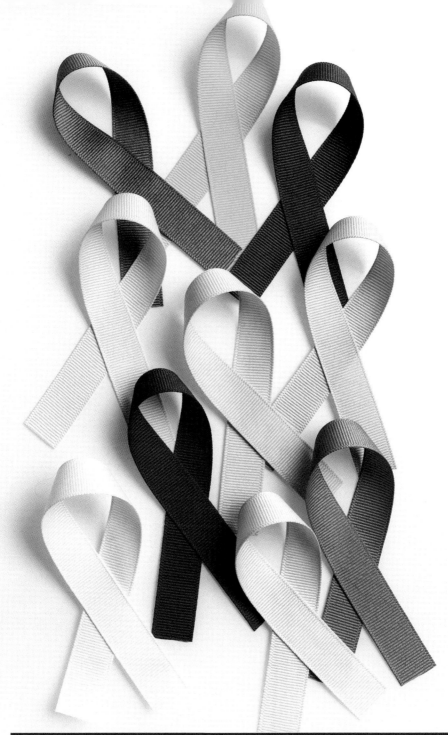

Cancer ribbons are loops of ribbon people wear to show support for those who have cancer or to spread awareness about cancer. Each color symbolizes a kind of cancer. For example, light blue stands for prostate cancer and pink means breast cancer.

GLOSSARY

anemia: Condition involving low red blood cell count.

benign: Noncancerous.

biopsy: The removal and examination of tissue for the purpose of diagnosis.

bone marrow: The spongy inner tissue of bones where blood cells are made.

cancer: General term for more than one hundred diseases in which abnormal cells grow out of control, damage healthy cells, and spread to other parts of the body.

carcinogen: A chemical or other substance that can cause cancer.

chemotherapy: Drugs and chemicals designed to kill cancer within the body.

clinical trial: An experimental study conducted on volunteers. Each study is designed to answer scientific questions and find new, better ways of preventing or treating cancer.

curative: Treatment aimed at bringing about a cure for cancer.

diagnosis: Identifying an illness or medical condition based on symptoms and exam.

gene: The basic unit of inheritance in a body's cells.

grade: A determination of how closely cancer cells resemble normal tissue; it is used to predict the rate at which cancer cells are likely to grow.

hormone: The natural substance released by an organ that influences the function of other organs in the body.

lymph nodes: Glands throughout the body that filter out harmful substances. Part of the immune system.

malignant: Cancerous.

metastasis: The spread of cancer from its first, or primary, tumor to other parts of the body.

oncogene: A gene that, when mutated or present at high levels, can help turn a normal cell into a cancer cell.

oncologist: A doctor who specializes in treating cancer.

pathologist: A doctor who specializes in the study of cells and tissues that have been removed from the body by biopsy or surgery.

platelet: The blood cell that helps stop bleeding by clotting at the wound.

predisposition: The state of being favorable or open to something beforehand; to have a tendency toward something.

radiation therapy: Cancer treatment with high-energy rays.

radiologist: A doctor specializing in the making of diagnostic medical images of areas inside the body. The images are made with X-rays, sound waves, and other types of energy.

recurrence: Regrowth of cancer cells after previous successful treatment.

red blood cell: The blood cell that supplies oxygen to tissues of the body.

remission: Temporary or permanent eradication of cancer cells from the body.

sarcoma: A cancer of the connective tissue of the body, such as bone and cartilage.

stage: A classification of a patient's cancer that takes into account the location of the primary tumor, the size and number of tumors, the spread of cancer into lymph nodes, the cell type, the tumor grade, and the presence or absence of metastasis.

suppress: To prevent the development or expression of.

tumor: A mass of tissue composed of an abnormal growth of cells. Tumors can be benign or malignant.

tumor suppressor gene: A gene that slows or stops the growth of tumors.

white blood cell: The blood cell that fights infection.

FOR MORE INFORMATION

American Cancer Society (ACS)
250 Williams Street NW
Atlanta, GA 30303
(800) 227-2345
Website: www.cancer.org
Facebook & Instagram: @americancancersociety
Twitter: @americancancer
The American Cancer Society is a nationwide organization committed to freeing the world from cancer. The group funds and conducts research, supports patients, and works to spread vital information about cancer prevention.

Canadian Cancer Society
55 St. Clair Avenue West, Ste. 500
Toronto, Ontario M4V 2Y7
(888) 939-3333
Website: cancer.ca
Facebook: @CanadianCancerSociety
Instagram & Twitter: @cancersociety
The Canadian Cancer Society is a national, community-based organization dedicated to improving and saving the lives of cancer patients through education, research, and advocacy.

Health Canada
Address Locator 0900C2
Ottawa, ON, K1A 0K9
Canada
(866) 225-0709

Website: www.hc-sc.gc.ca
The Canadian government is dedicated to informing its citizens about healthy living through info-
graphics and other resources. Funding opportunities are also available for grants and research.

Mayo Clinic
200 First Street SW
Rochester, MN 55905
(507) 284-2511
Website: www.mayoclinic.org
Facebook & Twitter: @MayoClinic
Each year more than one million patients seek
care at one of the three Mayo Clinic locations
across the United States. Known for their state-
of-the-art treatments, cutting edge research, and
helpful website resources.

Memorial Sloan Kettering Cancer Center
1275 York Avenue
New York, NY 10065
(800) 525-2225
Website: www.mskcc.org
Facebook & Instagram: @memorialsloankettering
Twitter: @sloan_kettering
The world's oldest and largest private cancer
center, Memorial Sloan Kettering has spent more
than 130 years devoted to innovative research,
exceptional patient care, and cutting-edge
research. Founded in 1884, the hospital is also
involved in community outreach.

National Cancer Institute (NCI)
9609 Medical Center Drive
Building 9609 MSC 9760
Bethesda, MD 20892
(800) 422-6237
Website: www.cancer.gov
Facebook: @cancer.gov
Twitter: @theNCI
Instagram: @nationalcancerinstitute/
Part of the United States' National Institutes
of Health, the National Cancer Institute is the
nation's leader in cancer research. Information on
diagnostics, treatment, clinical trials, and more
are available.

Teen Cancer America
11845 West Olympic Blvd.
Los Angeles, CA 90064
Website: teencanceramerica.org/
Facebook & Instagram: @TeenCancerAmerica
Twitter: @teencancerusa
Dedicated to improving the care options and
outcomes for teen cancer patients, this charity
was founded by musicians Roger Daltrey and Pete
Townshend. Programs include creating young
adult spaces at hospitals nationwide and other
support services for teens suffering from cancer.

FOR FURTHER READING

Brezina, Corona. *Cancer*. New York, NY: Rosen Publishing, 2021.

Charaipotra, Sona. *Symptoms of a Heartbreak*. New York, NY: Imprint, 2019.

Hand, Carol. *What You Need to Know About Health Insurance*. New York, NY: Rosen Publishing, 2020.

Hurt, Avery E. *Coping with Depression*. New York, NY: Rosen Publishing, 2020.

Murphy, Julie. *Side Effects May Vary*. New York, NY: Balzer + Bray, 2020. Print.

New York Times Educational Publishing. *Health Tech: The Apps and Gadgets Redefining Wellness*. New York, NY, New York Times Educational Publishing, 2019.

Rosenberg, Stephen A. *Overcome the Challenges of Cancer Care: How to Avoid Pitfalls on the Path to Healing*. Lanham, MD: Rowman & Littlefield, 2020.

Silver, Maya, and Marc Silver. *My Parent Has Cancer and It Really Sucks*. Naperville, IL: Sourcebooks, 2013.

Sonnenblick, Jordan. *Drums, Girls & Dangerous Pie*. Waterville, Maine: Thorndike Press, a part of Gale, a Cengage Company, 2020.

Thompson, Elissa. *James Till and Ernest McCulloch: The Team That Discovered Stem Cells*. New York, NY: Rosen Publishing, 2021.

INDEX

A
alcohol, 25, 30, 31
American Cancer Society, 4, 7, 28, 54

B
biological therapy, 76, 77
biopsy, 44, 69
bone marrow, 12, 17, 48, 77, 78
BRCA gene mutation, 27

C
carcinogen, 19, 22, 23, 24, 25, 27
Centers for Disease Control and Prevention (CDC),
    25, 35
chemotherapy, 73, 74, 75, 76, 77, 78
clinical trial, 82, 83
counseling, 53, 61, 62, 64, 85, 93

D
DNA, 18, 19, 22, 71

E
emotion, 50-61, 85, 86, 93

G
genetic, 9, 18-22, 26, 27

H
Hodgkin's lymphoma, 4, 6
human papillomavirus (HPV), 21, 26, 36

I
immune system, 13, 14, 16, 17, 22, 55, 76, 79, 80, 81
immunotherapy, 76, 77

L
leukemia, 12, 48
lymph nodes, 4, 13, 14, 15, 17, 40, 42, 49, 67, 71

lymphoma, 13

M
metastasis, 12, 67, 68
mole, 10, 32, 42

N
National Cancer Institute, 15, 25, 26, 36

O
oncogenes, 18, 19

R
radiation, 19, 69, 71, 72, 73, 77, 78
remission, 84, 85, 87

S
smoking, 24, 35
stages, 67, 68
stem cell transplant, 77, 78
surgery, 10, 39, 69, 70, 71, 79

T
tumor suppressor genes, 18, 19, 21

U
ultrasound, 46, 47
ultraviolet light, 23, 26, 32, 33

V
virus, 21, 26, 73

W
white blood cells, 16, 73, 76, 80

X
X-ray, 45, 46, 48

ABOUT THE AUTHOR

Elissa Bongiorno is a journalist who has been published in *USA Weekend*, the *Baltimore Sun*, and *In Touch Weekly*, among other publications. She received her master's in journalism from the University of Maryland and has written more than a dozen other titles for students, including *Coping with Stress, Coping with HIV/AIDS*, and *James Till and Ernest McCulloch: The Team That Discovered Stem Cells.*

CREDITS